# Social Problems in Cancer Control

# Social Problems in Cancer Control

Howard P. Greenwald
*Research Scientist*
*Battelle Human Affairs Research Centers*

**Ballinger Publishing Company** ● **Cambridge, Massachusetts**
*A Subsidiary of Harper & Row, Publishers, Inc.*

International Standard Book Number: ISBN 0-88410-708-6

Library of Congress Catalog Card Number: 79-15385

Printed in the United States of America

Library of Congress Cataloging in Publication Data

Greenwald, Howard P
Social Problems in Cancer Control
1. Cancer—Social aspects. 2. Cancer education—United States. 3. Health planning—United States. I. Title. [DNLM: 1. Health Planning. 2. Behavior. 3. Neoplasms—Prevention and control. QZ200.3 G816o]
RC262.G735                    362.1'9'699400973                    79-15385
ISBN 0-88410-708-6

# Contents

# List of Figures

# List of Tables

# Preface

This book represents a sociological contribution to health planning. As such, it hopes to provide a counterweight to a growing preoccupation in the minds of policymakers with the impersonal. Modern planning activities seem to draw more and more heavily on concrete, quantifiable matter such as budgets and legislative mandates. Analysis seems to focus increasingly on economics and econometrics, searching for explanations of policy outcomes in flows of capital and variations in purchasing power. Although the following chapters do not deny the importance of these perspectives, they do urge the reader to realize that neither the economy nor the law automatically affects human behavior. Policies and plans depend for success on the ability and willingness of actual persons to carry out their provisions. In a specialized but highly significant context, the control of cancer, this book attempts to demonstrate the importance of interpersonal and organizational factors even in the presence of abundant material resources and clear legislative direction. If legal and material entities represent "anatomical" constraints on policymaking, social relations reflect "physiological" realities. As in organic disease, an understanding of both factors is crucial to effective intervention.

The approach that is taken in this volume to problems in cancer control may differ from predominant tendencies in the behavioral sciences themselves. Although the analysis makes use of statistics, it uses numbers for essentially demonstrative purposes. Instead of discovering parameters representative of health professionals everywhere, it strives for an understanding of factors that affect their

ability to detect and treat cancer in a single geographic locality. Instead of developing mathematical models, it attempts to implant a
perspective in the mind of the reader. In its approach to empirical
date, the methodology used here sacrifices some degree of generaliz-
ability in the interests of comprehensibility. But the resulting trade-
off is quite compatible with the book's major goal: to suggest that
planners ask a general category of questions rather than provide them
with specific answers.

Who can benefit from this volume? It should be useful to anyone
occupying or contemplating entry into a planning role. Students in
health planning programs should find it useful in acquainting themselves with an important set of problems likely to emerge in many
specific contexts. Professional planners, even with a more rigorous
and quantitative orientation than this book follows, may learn a
good many specific facts about cancer and the problems of providing
care for other major health problems facing modern society. Beyond
these obvious categories, many other individuals such as physicians,
nurses, hospital administrators, social workers, and concerned members of the public may obtain valuable knowledge from this book. In
a sense, everybody today is a planner. Almost everyone can exert at
least a small amount of influence over resource allocation and the implementation of policy through his or her activities as a professional
or citizen. It is to this broad audience that the present volume speaks.

Howard Greenwald
Seattle, 1979

# Acknowledgments

I wish to thank a number of individuals for providing data, impressions, and assitance in this work. The National Cancer Institute, U.S. Department of Health, Education, and Welfare, provided initial funding for the study under grant no. NCI DHEW IR18 CA16401. The University of Chicago Center for Health Administration Studies, where this book was written, contributed additional resources. Dr. John E. Ultmann lent considerable encouragement and expertise to the project. June M. Smith and Erna L.K. Beaver contributed the major effort in design and administration of the Professional Community Survey. Selwyn W. Becker, Marshall D. Rosman, Robert L. Campbell, and Amanda Harmeling deserve credit for making major contributions to the project on noncompliance in cancer screening. Mrs. Adele Henrichsen of the American Cancer Society provided many valuable insights into the types of services most important to cancer patients and their families. Dr. Mary Marzotto of Northeastern Illinois State University added much to our understanding of community organizations and their concern for cancer detection and treatment. Many physicians, nurses, and other hospital personnel generously contributed their time to answer our questions. Barbara Hildebrand, R.N., M.S.N., added to our understanding of the nursing role. Michael Nevitt, Michael Donnelly, John Woodward, and David Berg provided much needed assistance and many ideas. Jane Grant, Edward H. Yelin, Elihu M. Gerson, Carl Milofsky, and Kitty Voss provided useful criticism of earlier drafts. Cindy Ostroff and Tanya Dusek-Gellen designed and executed the maps of Central City. Finally, the typists who prepared this and several earlier drafts deserve special recognition. Although they have become too numerous to mention individually, my debt to them is considerable.

# Social Problems in Cancer Control

# Chapter 1

# The Problem of Cancer Control

Cancer has long dominated the health concerns of Americans. Reflecting this concern, Congress earmarked greater and greater sums throughout the post-World War II era for research into the scientific and medical mysteries surrounding the disease. But during the 1960s policymakers began to adopt a new approach. As if to express increasing doubt that pure science could alone improve the lives of ordinary citizens, they shifted their attention from the laboratory to the doctor's office. Those concerned with reducing the death rate from cancer and other major health threats focused increasingly on the need to improve actual delivery of health care services and to promote wider application of advanced technology. As early as 1964, President Lyndon Johnson declared in a message to Congress:

> The Public Health Service is now spending well over a quarter of a billion dollars annually finding ways to combat [cancer, heart disease, and strokes]. . . . The flow of new discoveries, new drugs and techniques, is impressive and hopeful. Much remains to be learned. But the American people are not receiving the full benefit of what medical research has already accomplished.[1]

As if to echo President Johnson's confidence in the promise of more efficient health care delivery, a commission headed by Dr. Michael DeBakey concluded that "(many) things can be done now, without further scientific advance."[2]

From this perspective emerged the concept of "cancel control."

A program established under the National Cancer Act of 1971, the basic purpose of cancer control was to insure the rapid translation of new knowledge from the research laboratory into the treatment of the cancer patient, with the aim of reducing morbidity and mortality from the disease.[3] Supporters of the National Cancer Act often expressed unqualified optimism. President Richard M. Nixon, for example, characterized the legislation as "the most significant action" taken during his administration.[4] And a distinguished panel of consultants reporting to the Senate on the need for action against cancer promised that the five-year survival rate among cancer patients could be increased from one in three to one in two if the best techniques of diagnosis and treatment were made widely available.[5]

The National Cancer Act of 1971 formulated several specific goals for cancer control and made funds available for their implementation. Dr. D.J. Fink, Director of the National Cancer Institute's Division of Cancer Control and Rehabilitation, later summarized these aims.[6] According to Fink, the most prominent goals included: (1) insuring that "Practical and effective methods and techniques" of cancer prevention were available to and utilized by the public and health professionals; (2) promoting the continuing assessment of current practices and the development of principles for the optimal diagnoses and pretreatment evaluation of cancer patients; (3) insuring that practical and effective cancer screening and detection methods and techniques were available and utilized by populations at risk; and (4) aiding the development of principles and facilities for the optimal treatment, rehabilitation, and continuing care of cancer patients. Provisions of the act encouraged the integration of research and patient care. In addition, recognizing that implementation of these goals would require greatly enhanced coordination among divergent parts of the health care system, a series of amendments specified that grants an contracts awarded under the act should promote cooperative efforts among hospitals, physicians, public health departments, and voluntary organizations.[7]

Though highly attractive to both politicians and the public, cancer control presents a series of vexing dilemmas to health planners. Technical means may indeed exist that could save many lives if more widely applied by physicians, nurses, and other health care providers. But the pattern of social relationships that characterizes health care in the contemporary United States makes achievement of this goal extremely difficult. Any significant degree of success in cancer control would require transformations in the relations among physicians, between physicians and other health professionals, among organizations providing health care services, and between health care providers and the public. The capacity of planners to help control cancer will depend on their comprehension of these relations and ability to help change them.

This book is a sociological analysis of interrelations among individuals involved in the detection and treatment of cancer, beliefs about cancer and its management, and allocation of resources to fight cancer. It provides planners with examples of ways in which social relations affect cancer control activities. Instead of attempting an exhaustive study of a single aspect of cancer control, this volume treats several loosely related issues in an illustrative manner. It is hoped that this strategy will encourage readers to develop a sufficiently general perspective to apply in instances they themselves encounter that are not covered by this or any other study of health care.

The problems involved in successfully controlling cancer appear most clearly when contrasted with mankind's earlier attempts to control disease. The work of Walter Reed and his associates, for example, is well known, and Paul de Kruif's history of the conquest of yellow fever has doubtlessly helped mold the career decision of many a modern health professional. But a brief look at the De Kruif narrative illustrates its inappropriateness as a paradigm for disease control today. DeKruif indicates, for instance, that the part that Stegomyia mosquitoes played in the spread of yellow fever was easily established through a single and quite straightforward experimental procedure:

> Clad only in a nightshirt and fresh from a bath (a volunteer) walked into the healthy little room and lay down on his clean cot. In a minute, that damned buzzing started around his head, in two minutes he was bitten, in the thirty minutes he lay there he was stabbed seven times—without even the satisfaction of smashing those mosquitoes. . . . He was back at four-thirty the same afternoon, to be bitten again . . . .
>
> On Christmas morning of 1900, there was a fine present waiting for him—in his head, how that thumped—in his eyes, how red they were and how the light hurt them—in his bones, how tired they were! . . . So at last Walter Reed had every answer to his diabolical question, and he wrote, in that old-fashioned prose of his: "The essential factor in the infection of a building with yellow fever is the presence therein of mosquitoes that have bitten cases of yellow fever."[8]

Reed easily silenced those who disputed his findings:

> But still there came learned doctors . . . from Europe and America . . . asking this, questioning that . . . . "These are remarkable experiments,

but the results should be weighed and considered with reserve . . . et cetera!" Then the gauze lid came off a jar of she-mosquitoes (of course it was by accident) and into the room, with wicked lustful eyes on those learned scientists the Stegomyia buzzed. Alas for skepticism! Away with all doubts! From the room rushed the eminent savants of knowledge! Down went the screen door with a crash—such was the vehemence of their conviction that Walter Reed was right.[9]

Application of the discovery was rapid and the results dramatic:

William Crawford Gorgas . . . went into the gutters and cesspools and cisterns of Habana, making horrid war on the Stegomyia mosquitoes, and in ninety days, Habana had not a single case of yellow jack—she was free for the first time in two hundred years. It was magical![10]

All this, according to DeKruif's history, was accomplished through the efforts of a handful of brave and dedicated innovators using highly simple techniques.

Many problems face those seeking to control cancer that were absent in the work of Walter Reed and other fighters of infectious disease. The understanding of cancer that scientists now possess may well be less complete than the understanding their counterparts in the early 1900s possessed of infectious disease. Medical approaches to cancer detection and treatment are far from standardized in contemporary practice and scientific discourse. The efficacy of even the most fundamental cancer control procedures such as early detection remain subjects of vigorous debate.[11] In the absence of a widely accepted theory of the diffusion of cancer, control efforts have focused on efficient detection and treatment rather than reducing incidence in the classic public health tradition. This feature of cancer control adds greatly to the complexity of the task. Cancer patients differ widely among themselves; patients may need several different types of care, the requirements for one case seldom duplicating those of any other. Cancer control, then, appears to depend on the efforts of numerous professionals treating clinically complex ailments whose characteristics differ markedly from patient to patient.

The cancer control procedures outlined by the National Cancer Act are clearly less dramatic than those described by DeKruif. In comparison, the process of providing the patient with the most appropriate care as rapidly as possible—either through instruction of local health professionals or transferring patients to the care of more expert practitioners—sounds burdensome and mundane. Yet this approach may be highly reasonable given the existing state of cancer-fighting technology available to the medical profession. The methods of cancer control outlined above, for example, appear cheap in comparison to the gigantic expenditures devoted in the past to hospital construction and basic research. A regional cancer control program could consist primarily of educational efforts. Such an effort would involve neither "brick and mortar" construction of new facilities nor major financial and administrative innovations among health care providers. It might aim specifically at developing a strong local cadre of competent professional personnel specialized in oncology and active referral relationships among physicians at community hospitals and a university-based referral center. Such a program could include educational outreach by university medical school faculty to community physicians through their hospitals. It might offer special courses and training seminars in oncology for community nurses. Such instruction would be valuable to community practitioners, many of whom may have found their professional lives too active to keep up with recent developments in cancer diagnosis and therapy. All these activities could help actual cancer patients more than costly construction or lengthy research endeavors.

But activity of this kind cannot continue for long on a scale of any significance in the absence of adequate *social technology*. All technical activity requires patterns of social relations that allow the activity to take place. Social technology encompasses the habits, customs, and institutions that support concrete activity, whether economic, scientific, or medical in nature. In science, for example, little progress could take place without the existence of universities, the financial support of researchers, the widespread diffusion of knowledge through learned journals and scholarly conventions, and the belief among scientists that discoveries should be shared with colleagues.[12] The modern firm requires a social technology that differs markedly from the family unit in agrarian society. No large factories could be built, no automobiles or penicillin produced in the absence of contractual relationships to reduce the uncertainty of economic activity or respect among workers for the authority of individuals outside their families. Similarly, effective cancer control cannot take place in a medical community lacking values and norms that encourage the widespread diffusion of complex knowledge, the convenient transfer of patients from the care of one practitioner to another, or the sharing of responsibilities among physicians and other categories of health professionals.

While medical technology may have developed far enough to provide many cancer victims with more effective care than they now receive, the social technology that prevails among health care providers today appears fundamentally inadequate to translate improved medical knowledge into better patient services. Just as the modern firm requires employees to accept modes of work discipline substantially different from agrarian society, an effective cancer control program requires major departures from the method by which health care providers have traditionally dispensed their services. Although physicians have hitherto relied on patients to approach them when they experienced the physical discomfort that accompanies disease, the medical community must take more positive steps toward early detection. While the traditional practice of medicine has typically stressed individual physician competence and responsibility for the patient, the idea of cancer control requires greater coordination, sharing of knowledge, increased consultation among practitioners, and stronger, more frequently used referral relationships. While health care in the United States has become increasingly technical and specialized in the late twentieth century, meaningful control of cancer requires that health care providers make a broad range of services including such intangibles as emotional support available to patients. And although nurses and other nonphysician health professionals have been relegated to standardized, routine activities in the past, they must now receive encouragement to continue learning and exercise greater professional responsibilities. Unless researchers discover a miraculous cure for all varieties of cancer in the near future—a treatment, moreover, that need be administered only once and has no side effects—ameliorating the effects of cancer on the U.S. population will require changes in health care delivery along these lines.

This book provides the planner with a detailed understanding of the gap between the social technology presently employed in cancer detection and treatment and the social technology necessary for effective cancer control. It first specifies the range of needs that health care providers must address if they are to adequately serve cancer patients or others threatened or affected by the disease. Second, it examines the supply of resources available for cancer control in a specific locality and the manner in which these resources are distributed within the region. Third, it presents a detailed picture of the organization of professionals specialized in fighting cancer and identifies factors that represent barriers to necessary change. Fourth, it demonstrates the effects of interrelations among cancer-oriented professionals and between these professionals and the public upon the ability of the health care system to perform several important cancer-related functions. Finally, it connects specific issues related to cancer control with general problems in the health care system and suggests concrete planning strategies for improving the system's capacity to deal with cancer.

The chapters that follow address these issues by examining the experiences of an actual cancer control program. Active between 1974 and 1977, this program was organized as an adjunct to the cancer research activities of a major university medical center. Its goals, largely educational in nature, closely followed the guidelines of the National Cancer Act. Concretely, they included (1) a tumor registry program, designed to create a central depository of information on cancer cases for purposes including studies of management and outcome; (2) a nursing oncology program, which offered nurses in the locale courses in such subjects as the basic concepts of chemotherapy and radiation therapy, pediatric oncology, and psychosocial management of cancer patients; and (3) educational outreach programs for community physicians in oncology via visits by university faculty to community hospital conferences. Like the National Cancer Act itself, the program's directors expressed optimistic goals:

> We believe that these efforts will result in providing advanced cancer diagnosis and therapy to patients in the region while establishing a network of referral, properly utilizing the best professional talent available for the benefit of the public.

The program included an effort to estimate the needs, resources, and problems related to cancer detection and treatment in the surrounding region. This component of the cancer control effort generated most of the data on which the present volume is based. Research in this area took place in several ways. First, and most important, were conversations with the organizers of the program as well as health care professionals throughout the region. Second, the book includes findings from a survey of the local professional community (designated in the text as the Professional Community Survey), which sampled the opinions of 413 health care professionals and outpatients undergoing radiation therapy for the treatment of cancer. Third, the discussion below makes use of a survey of services and attitudes held by local public agencies and community groups toward the aims of cancer control. Finally, the volume presents findings from a study of the attitudes of individuals undergoing screening for the early detection of cancer at a facility specialized in this function. A full discussion of research methods and sampling procedures is in the appendix.

Throughout the book, the discussion concentrates upon the patterns of relationships among professionals and between the public and the health care system. Earlier studies have approached this problem from several diverse perspectives. Strauss and his associates, for example, have conducted highly detailed studies of the interactions among professionals and between professionals and patients in the care of cancer and other serious diseases. These researchers have achieved a high degree of intimacy with the problems of serious illness, effectively providing readers with an understanding of the social processes that prevail in treatment. This research reveals intricate patterns of behavior such as complex and often implicit bargaining by which participants strive to enhance their autonomy and protect the quality of their lives. The writings of Strauss and his group provide extremely powerful illustrations of the emotional stresses that often characterize life-threatening disease.[13]

From a much broader perspective, another group of researchers focuses on the structure of the health care system as a whole to explain the problems faced by patients and professionals alike. Alford, for example, attributes the major problems in health care to "the existence of a network of political, legal, and economic institutions which guarantees that certain dominant interests will be served."[14] According to this reasoning, the inability of the health care system to effectively control cancer would follow in part from the fact that powerful groups in contemporary American society such as physicians place more importance on protection of their privileged positions than meeting social needs.

The present volume disputes neither of these two perspectives. It aims instead at adding to the understanding of management of serious illness that they have already provided. The present study focuses on phenomena that are more abstract than the intimate perspective of Strauss and more concrete than Alford's broad view. This book provides a close look at selected features of cancer detection and treatment in a particular geographical region in hopes of establishing the existence of patterns that are likely to be present throughout the United States. While the findings presented here may at times overlap with Strauss and Alford, the need for a complete understanding of problems in cancer control is great enough to permit occasional restatement of already established themes. Instead of merely repeating these themes, furthermore, the present study adds quantitative support for findings that Strauss presents in a discursive manner and provides specific examples of principles Alford states in broad and usually abstract language.

This book employs an approach to the structure and organization of cancer-related services considerably less formal than the tools employed by the management scientist. Planners today often find techniques such as operations research attractive because they approach health-related issues in a systematic and explicit fashion. Operations research techniques allow analysts to construct models of specifiable inputs and outputs among parts of industrial plants, business organizations, or hospitals. Corporate planners often find operations research highly useful in reorganizing a department for the purpose of maximizing unidimensional and quantifiable outcomes such as the profits of a firm.[15] Critics of operations research, though, have argued that it is considerably less useful in dealing with more general planning problems. Hoos, for example, points out that the applicability of operations research is quite limited in cases where outcome standards are subject to dispute or several different outcomes may be of equal value.[16] While operations research and similar techniques may assist the hospital administrator in coordinating the needs of various departments, they do not help the planner understand the factors that promote such difficult to quantify "products" as high-quality emotional support for terminal cancer patients or such elusive matters as the appropriate application of complex medical technology to cancer cases. Because its relative informality permits an examination of several distinct factors that together promote or inhibit successful cancer control efforts, the approach taken in the present study contributes an understanding not normally available through management science.

Readers may still object that effective control of cancer requires more "scientific" methods than those appearing in this volume. Readers who are biomedically oriented, for example, may argue that nothing of any importance can be achieved without a basic understanding of the cause of cancer. Those subscribing to public health or political perspectives may contend that cancer control efforts should concentrate on identifying carcinogenic industrial products and ridding the environment of them. Believers in the continuing independence of community medicine may dispute the implication that highly specialized practitioners and doctors at academic medical centers can treat cancer more successfully than family physicians.

All of these caveats have significant bases in fact. Leading epidemiologists have argued, for example, that the vast majority of all human cancers are attributable to environmental carcinogens such as radioactive substances and food additives.[17] A comprehensive review of literature on several medical specialties has revealed no consistent relationship between board certification (an indication of degree of specialization) and quality of care.[18] And biomedical researchers can safely argue that cancer deaths will never be reduced to a minimum before the disease's etiology and biochemical features are fully understood.

But despite these realities, cancer control as outlined above must remain a vital national priority. Because cancer is such a prevalent cause of death in the modern world, even a slight increase in the survival rate translates into additional years of life for numerous individuals. Assuming that even a small fraction of the discoveries recently made by cancer researchers are immediately applicable in community medical practice, numerous lives can be saved and the lives of cancer victims beyond the possibility of cure can be made more comfortable. Lack of complete knowledge of the cause of yellow fever did not induce Walter Reed to delay beginning control measures that immediately reduced mortality.[19] The isolation of environmental carcinogens may have little effect as the public continues to demand their availability (as occurred with saccharin) and industries require their use for efficient production. Even though specialists may be no better able to treat some forms of cancer than community physicians, patients with at least some malignancies stand a better chance of survival at major referral centers than in local community hospitals. A study of colon cancer in Illinois by the American Cancer Society, for example, reveals that patients with Stage III malignancies (indicating invasion of immediately adjacent organs) survived for five years after diagnosis over 66 percent of the time at a major academic center in Chicago, but only 16, 17, and 22 percent of the time at hospitals in Peoria, Belleville, and Rockford, respectively.[20]

This introduction has attempted to alert the reader to the relevance of social factors to effective cancer control given the level of medical technology in the late twentieth century. The remainder of the book will provide specific illustrations of the effect of social relations on cancer control activities and set forth general policy implications. Chapter 2 specifies the needs that the health care system must meet if it is to effectively address the threat of cancer and draws implications from cancer for other serious threats to health in modern society. Chapter 3 provides a detailed description of an actual cancer control program and the characteristics of the region in which it operates. This chapter is intended to illustrate the concrete tasks of a regional cancer control program. Chapter 4 deals with the physician community, a key element in the success or failure of any health planning effort. This chapter discusses the interpersonal and traditional features of the medical profession, asking whether they stand in the way of improved information flow and patient referral among practitioners. Chapter 5 describes the pattern of relationships between doctors and other health care workers, asking whether the authority relations on the health care team inhibit or promote the aims of cancer control. Chapter 6 considers the problem of emotional support for cancer patients, asking whether the organization of the health care team is optimally effective in providing this important service. Chapter 7 examines the early detection process. It asks which segments of the population are most and least likely to seek regular, early detection for cancer, which factors may inhibit those who seek cancer screening from gaining the full benefits of the procedure, and how early detection facilities can be integrated into the health care system to insure the most rapid and effective movement of patients suspected of having cancer to treatment sites. Chapter 8 draws general policy implications from the preceding chapters and makes suggestions for implementing the goals of cancer control and similar heath care programs. The appendix contains copies of the research instruments that generated data for this book and discusses the research methodology used to analyze the data.

## NOTES

1. Lyndon B. Johnson, "Special Message to the Congress on the Nation's Health," February 10, 1964, U.S. President, *Public Papers of the President: Lyndon B. Johnson*, 1963-64, vol. 1, Washington, D.C.: U.S. Government Printing Office, 1965, p. 282.

2. President's Commission on Heart Disease, Cancer, and Stroke, *Report to the President: A National Program to Conquer Heart Disease, Cancer, and Stroke*, vol. 1, Washington, D.C.: U.S. Government Printing Office, December 1964, p. xi.

3. Richard A. Rettig, *Cancer Crusade: The Story of the National Cancer Act of 1971* (Princeton: Princeton University Press, 1977), p. 303.

4. Ibid., p. 277.

5. Ibid., p. 303.

6. Diane J. Fink, "The Cancer Control Program," *Cancer* 35 (May 1975): 71-75.

7. Ibid.

8. Paul DeKruif, *Microbe Hunters* (New York: Harcourt, Brace and Company, 1926), p. 328.

9. Ibid., pp. 329-330.

10. Ibid., p. 329.

11. David Sacket, "Periodic Examination of Patients at Risk," in D. Schottenfeld, ed., *Cancer Epidemiology and Prevention* (Springfield, Ill.: Charles C. Thomas, 1975).

12. Robert K. Merton, *Social Theory and Social Structure* (New York: The Free Press, 1964), p. 556.

13. An excellent example of this research tradition is Barney Glazer and Anselm Strauss, *Awareness of Dying* (Chicago: Aldine Publishing Co., 1965).

14. Robert R. Alford, *Health Care Politics* (Chicago: University of Chicago Press, 1975), p. 17.

15. Russell L. Ackoff and Maurice W. Sasieni, *Fundamentals of Operations Research* (New York: John Wiley, 1968). See Chapter 17.

16. Ida R. Hoos, *Systems Analysis and Public Policy—A Critique* (Berkeley: University of California Press, 1972), pp. 140-141.

17. P.B. Medawar, "The Crab," *New York Review of Books* 24 (June 9, 1977), p. 11.

18. K.N. Williams and R.H. Brook, "Quality Measurement and Assurance," *Health and Medical Care Sciences Review* 1 (May/June 1978), pp. 1-12.

19. DeKruif, op. cit., pp. 330-333.

20. American Cancer Society, *Results in Treating Cancer, Report No. 2: Colon Cancer* (Chicago: American Cancer Society, 1977), pp. 12-13.

# Chapter 2

# Cancer and the Health Care System

This chapter provides a detailed examination of the functions that the health care system must perform if it is to reduce the threat of cancer in contemporary America. An understanding of these tasks must precede consideration of the organizational patterns and social processes that interefere with their performance. The management of cancer must take place in ways quite distinct from many other diseases. But cancer poses problems that typify the most important health care problems facing modern society. An account of the specific needs that the health care system must meet to aid individuals faced with cancer poses central issues for the system as a whole, raising the disturbing possibility that the basic traditions of health care and the method by which it is organized in twentieth-century America are incompatible with the needs of today's society.

The objective of this study is, once again, the determination of social realities that contradict the capacity of the health care system to mitigate the threat of cancer in modern society by reducing mortality from the disease and limiting its disruptive influences on the lives of its victims and their families. The book's perspective generally looks beyond the problems of individuals stricken with cancer, searching instead for the roots of individual problems within the social system surrounding health care. But the gravity of cancer's effects on the lives of individuals is too great to risk losing sight of this dimension in the pursuit of "social facts." Because only the personal aspects of cancer can remind the analyst of the concrete importance of the general issues considered here, it seems essential to begin by couching the problems that the disease creates in individual terms.

For example, consider the thoughts of a middle-aged woman as she leaves a modern, low-rise building somewhere in the Midwest. She is worried, perhaps more than ever before in her life. Her anxiety is easy to understand. Her physician, whose office she has just left, has informed her that she may be seriously ill. Although he did not specify the disorder he suspected, he hinted strongly at cancer. He used words like "suspicious cells" and "dangerous growth." These words were disturbingly familiar. She had heard them used years earlier when her mother had entered a hospital, later dying of cancer. She wonders, "Is it my turn now?"

She had expected nothing particularly unusual to occur. Having noticed an abnormal discharge from her vagina about two weeks earlier, she had made the appointment for strictly precautionary purposes. Although slightly alarmed at the time, she had calmed herself. She recognized in herself a tendency to magnify the importance of minor abnormalities. Nevertheless, she telephoned her doctor's office without delay. One could never be too careful, and what were doctors for, anyway? Her family belonged to a prepaid health care plan covering most medical services, and thus the precautionary visit would cost nothing extra. It made complete sense.

But the encounter with her physician had been a nightmare. He had given her a quick pelvic examination, performed a few other seemingly routine procedures, and made some notes on her chart. Then he left the room, returning after a few moments with another doctor. The second physician felt carefully around her midsection, seeming to know exactly where to place his fingers. Then both doctors left, giving her time to dress. Her own physician reappeared shortly, seating himself at his desk and motioning to her to take a seat nearby. Then he had begun to explain about a mass that would need surgical exploration. He never used the word "cancer." Still the firmness and urgency in his voice suggested something grave. She could feel a throbbing in her throat and a tingling sensation on her skin when he announced that he was admitting her to the hospital and immediately began filling out the necessary forms. The doctor stressed that he was admitting her for exploratory surgery only, and could make no diagnosis before the surgeons had done their work. But in spite of these disclaimers, she felt more frightened than on any occasion she could recall. Although the doctor had chosen his language carefully, using words like "exploratory" and "precautionary," all she remembered were "suspicious mass," "hospitalization," and "surgery."

Back on the street, she wonders what to do first. Should she call her husband at work, or wait for him to return home to break the news? Should she go home and prepare for her trip to the hospital, scheduled for the next morning? Should she try to find someone to talk with, compare experiences, and help alleviate her anxiety? Should she telephone her two sons, neither of whom lives at home, to tell them the news? Orienting herself to the concrete necessities of the moment, she heads for the parking lot.

She decides to go home. Her thoughts run from the immediate to the remote, from the realistic to the fanciful, from the critical to the trivial as she drives. She wonders whether she will live or die. She had heard that medicine has made "tremendous strides" against cancer in recent years, yet she knows several people who have died from the disease, one living his last months in extreme pain and fear. She asks herself, "Who's going to watch the house while I'm in the hospital?" She tries to recall the details of her family medical insurance package, realizing that although it appears to cover everything, unanticipated expenses always seem to accompany hospitalization. She thinks about the financial needs of her sons, one of whom is employed but the other still in college. "How am I going to tell everyone?" she wonders, realizing that her husband, always the "nervous" type, does not handle crises well, and her sons are still "boys." For a fleeting moment, she considers a trip to Florida. "If I'm going to die," she reasons, "I might as well do it in a nice place. Why go to the hospital at all? They can't do anything for cancer."

This vignette illustrates some of the central problems associated with cancer that America's health care apparatus must approach effectively to mitigate the effect of cancer on human life. The experiences of the woman described above, first, are not unusual. The American Cancer Society estimated that in 1977 physicians would discover cancer in 700,000 Americans, and that 10 million would undergo treatment for the disease in the 1970s.[1] A proportionally vast segment of the nation's health care resources is devoted to the detection and treatment of cancer. Second, the dread that she experiences is quite common. While heart disease kills more Americans than all forms of cancer combined, cancer creates greater levels of fear in the lives of its victims and those close to them. Researchers note that cancer has a 47 percent curability rate, while 50 percent of all stroke sufferers die within one year of the stroke and 35 percent of all coronary victims succumb within a month of the heart attack.[2] The word "cancer" has a more intractable, awesome, and terrifying quality than diseases that are in fact much less readily managed by modern medicine. Perhaps most disconcerting is the observation that numerous physicians harbor attitudes toward cancer that are equally pessimistic. A major survey of physicians treating cancer in the 1960s revealed a widespread belief that doctors can "do very little to save lives and not a great deal to prevent suffering" among patients afflicted with the disease.[3]

Third, the fictional patient described above experiences a level of uncertainty that is highly typical of real cancer patients. Cancer can be a clinical entity that defies conclusive diagnosis and reliable prognosis. But, as with other serious illnesses,[4] physicians often do not disclose to patients that they have cancer even when the diagnosis is certain. Wishing to prevent their patients from losing hope and to avoid exposure to emotional outburst common among those informed that they have contracted life-threatening illnesses, doctors avoid terms like "cancer" and "malignancy" whenever possible. As McIntosh has observed, "The euphemistic content of their communication (enables) the doctors to avoid giving explicit information while, at the same time, not telling any lies."[5] While often motivated by humanitarian factors, nondisclosure has drawbacks as well. Numerous patients undoubtedly experience greater anxiety in the state of uncertainty than they would if they were told the real nature of their illness.

Whether the physician informs a patient directly of his or her malignacy or the patient infers the fact from informal cues gleaned during encounters with the health care system, severe emotional and social reprecussions are likely to result. In addition to extreme fear, cancer victims often experience "an inner revulsion, a concept of feeling themselves unclean."[6] The inexplicable and often unexpected discovery of cancer fills many patients with a sense of injustice, a temptation to ask the question, "Why me?"

Social estrangement and isolation often aggravate the cancer patient's emotional difficulties. Hospitalization and physical disability, of course, make it difficult for the patient to remain in contact with friends and relatives. Whether the malignancy ultimately proves curable or fatal, the interval between discovery and outcome is typically protracted and uncertain in length. The tension and uncertainty inherent in the cancer patient's career often create extreme levels of anxiety among friends and relatives. Those close to the patient may resent the demands he or she makes upon them for company and support. As a psychiatrist who specializes in the cancer patient's social and emotional problems has observed:

> When people believe that an illness is going to be terminal, they are literally waiting for the victim to die. . . . There is an unspoken anger and guilt

that follows. . . . The friend or relative of a cancer patient has to keep telling himself that he shouldn't be weary at all the visiting and traveling he has to do, (and) shouldn't be angry at all the fuss. . . .[7]

Although individuals in our society typically look to friends and relatives for support when they are seriously ill or sense the approach of death, personal intimates are often unable to meet the need. The experience of one cancer patient vividly illustrates this problem. Describing his experiences in the hospital, he recalled that his visitors often became more upset than he. "I would have to take care of *them*," he said.[8]

A great many of the problems that the cancer patient experiences on the psychological plane appear to arise from the cultural image of cancer in modern America. In a highly absorbing analysis, Susan Sontag describes this image as a disease "overlaid with mystification" and "charged with the fantasy of inescapable fatality."[9] Sontag notes that contemporary literature tends to omit many of the personally redeeming features connected with dread diseases of the past:

> While TB takes on qualities assigned to the lungs, which are part of the upper, spiritualized body, cancer is notorious for attacking parts of the body (colon, rectum, breast, cervix, prostate, testicles) that are embarrassing to acknowledge. . . . A disease of the lungs is, metaphorically, a disease of life. Cancer, a disease that can strike anywhere, is a disease of the body. Far from proving anything spiritual, it proves that the body is, alas, and all too much, the body.[10]

Sontag points out that popular theories that connect cancer with repressed emotions and major life disappointments give cancer victims an even more negative image:

> . . . there is mostly opprobrium attached to a disease thought to stem from the repression of emotion—an opprobrium echoed in the view of cancer propagated by Reich, and the many writers influenced by him. Reich's view of cancer as a disease of the failure of expressiveness condemns the cancer patient: expresses pity but also conveys contempt. The theory also contributes to making cancer shameful, and to making cancer patients feel, consciously or unconsciously, guilty for getting cancer.[11]

Sontag interprets this view of cancer as a mechanism by which the healthy distance themselves from the imperfections in modern technology that cancer represents and in the process blame the cancer victim for becoming ill.

The anxieties experienced by the fictional patient described above illustrate several concrete problems that the health care system must overcome if its efforts to control the devastating effects of cancer are to be effective. Beyond her need for a medical technology, capable of arresting, curing, or mitigating the discomfort of cancer, this patient requires assistance in adjusting emotionally to the life-threatening condition. She requires a health care system that communicates effectively with her about the nature of her illness and explains what she can expect to encounter when treatment begins. Her momentary doubt about the efficacy of medical treatment for cancer and fleeting temptation to withdraw from care suggests that many other patients with similar symptoms would need more active encouragement to seek diagnosis and therapy. The characteristics of her family imply that its members will not be able to furnish the emotional support she needs unaided. The suspicion that new expenses may arise from a hospital stay raises the very real issue that many in a similar position do not have sufficient coverage to survive catastrophic illness financially even if they recover physically.

But the problems raised by this woman's experience represent only a few of those that face a society intent upon ameliorating the effects of cancer upon its population. The fictional patient, for example, apparently possesses social advantages lacked by many others in the same metropolitan area. First, she has better initial access to the health care system than the average citizen. A member of a prepaid health care plan, she has a regular source of medical care, a resource not shared by a large number of her fellow Americans. She has a regular physician, who both knows her history and cares about her well-being, a phenomenon not to be taken for granted in a health maintenance organization. She is careful about her health, and she is sufficiently concerned about it to make a visit to the doctor for purely precautionary purposes. She has sufficient confidence in doctors and medical technology to willingly brave the uncertainties of hospitalization and surgery. Her physician has sufficient concern for his patients and understanding of the extremely fearful nature of cancer to begin hospital admission proceedings even before she has left his office, a tactic designed to make sure she complies with his recommendation of exploratory surgery. The patient has a family that, even if it cannot provide all the emotional support she needs, will provide some. She has a car, is able to drive it, can find parking near her doctor's office, and is unafraid to walk from her vehicle to the medical center.

Many of the woman's neighbors in the upper middle-class suburb in which she lives are as likely to contract cancer at some time in their lives as she. But some would encounter even greater difficulties in dealing with the disease. Those who are elderly may depend upon others for transportation, first to the doctor's office, and later, after surgery, to the hospital for follow-up treatment. They may not be fortunate enough to have relatives living close enough to provide them with company or emotional support. If they are less educated, they are relatively unlikely to utilize a doctor's services for precautionary purposes.[12] Even if they have been financially able to support an upper middle-class style of life, they may never have found a physician they returned to regularly, and lacking sufficient medical insurance, face extreme financial burdens.

A woman with the same medical condition would encounter many additional problems if she were poor and black. First, she would be less likely to have a regular source of medical care, and even if she had a customary site where she saw a doctor, she would probably not see the same physician at each visit.[13] She would be less likely to utilize medical services for preventive purposes than her white, comparatively affluent counterpart, and she would have less confidence in the ability of physicians to treat serious illness.[14] Transportation and physical safety getting to and from the doctor's office would pose greater problems for the poor black than the upper middle-class white woman. Because of racial and class differences, the black woman may encounter greater difficulty in communicating with the physician. Also because of these inhibiting factors, she would be more likely to postpone her visit to a physician after becoming aware of an alarming abnormality and less likely to follow up the initial visit. While most doctors are white males, the white female is not nearly as socially distant from the doctor, sharing his race and perhaps his class background. Ironically, the black is statistically more likely to need the quality and quantity of resources possessed by the white cancer patient. Blacks in the United States have a higher incidence of cancer than whites. Perhaps because they lack the resources related to health care available to whites, the death rate from cancer among blacks is also higher.

While serious, these problems represent only the most visible of those confronting the cancer patient. Returning to the middle-aged white woman who has just emerged from the doctor's office, what problems is she likely to face at future stages in her career as a cancer patient? First, many features of the hospital she enters may present additional difficulties. While her doctor's office may be conveniently located, the hospital to which she is admitted for exploratory surgery may not be. Wishing to place her in a position to receive the best possible medical care, the physician may admit her to a hospital in the city's central core. This location may be congested, limiting access by car and hence reducing the number of visits from family and friends. The area may have a reputation of being unsafe, which, deserved or undeserved, will have the same effect on visitation.

In the hospital, the patient will have to contend with a new set of discouraging dilemmas. First, she is likely to encounter difficulties in obtaining information both before and after the planned surgery. The interns and residents who ask her questions about her medical history and perform tests in preparation for surgery are likely to respond to her queries in vague generalities. The nurses, whom she will encounter more frequently than any other class of hospital personnel, will be caught up in a time-consuming routine of gathering medical data, unable to spend much time with her, and disinclined to answer questions about her case. She will have to undergo many uncomfortable testing procedures. Finally, a resident is likely to ask her for permission to allow the surgical team to remove any diseased tissue they may find in the exploratory procedure, obviating the necessity of a second operation, and request her to sign a legal document indicating consent. These typical characteristics of hospitalization will almost certainly increase the level of anxiety the patient began to experience at her doctor's office.

New difficulties will emerge following surgery. Assume, for example, that the surgeons discover a regionalized malignancy of the large intestine and perform a colostomy. This procedure will necessitate several types of follow-up care. The patient will need instruction in caring for the colostomy, as well as assistance in adjusting emotionally to radical alteration of a basic bodily function. In addition, she will require continuing radiation therapy, chemotherapy, or both. Numerous, regular return trips to the hospital will probably be necessary. The patient may no longer feel able to drive herself to the hospital and will have to depend on others for assistance. If the hospital at which she undergoes surgery does not provide all the follow-up services she needs, she may require referral to a distant site. All this activity may be accompanied by the discomfort—for many patients, extreme pain is a more accurate word—that often follows surgery and results from both radiation and chemotherapy. Finally, the patient will have to live with the constantly present possibility that her malignancy will recur despite treatment.

Perhaps the most important problems related to this woman's career as a cancer patient are those of which she will never be aware. Her doctor, for example, must make several important decisions about her case at the moment he realizes that she may have cancer.

He must decide, for example, whether he has the skill and experience necessary to handle the case himself, or whether it would be wiser to refer her to another physician. This dilemma will become more difficult at the postsurgical stage of the patient's career when the use of newly developed therapeutic drugs may require the knowledge of a specialist in oncology. The decision will become considerably more important if the disease recurs. At this point, the doctor may have to decide whether to readmit the patient to his own hospital, remaining the attending physician on the case, or refer the patient to a colleague with greater skills and knowledge and admitting privileges at a hospital with more advanced technical equipment and specialized personnel. At any time during the patient's illness the doctor must decide whether to ask the opinion of other physicians, perhaps taking the risk that his colleagues will interpret such action as an indication of incompetence or at least disinclination to keep up with the latest developments in cancer therapy. The pattern of professional relations in which the physician finds himself, his specialty, his education, his personality, and his financial needs will all play significant parts in his decision to consult other doctors or refer patients to them. The patient, of course, has no knowledge of this feature of medical practice. But it can easily determine whether or not she will survive her illness.

The dilemmas and reversals that this patient will encounter in her struggle with cancer are not hers alone. They do not arise from flaws in her personality or malice among other human beings. Every physician, nurse, and technician she meets, for example, may genuinely wish to give her the best possible care. Volunteer groups with the most humane motives may do their best to provide auxiliary services in such areas as emotional support and transportation. Lawmakers may throw the massive resources of government behind efforts to find a cancer cure at least in part owing to humane motives. Yet the health professionals she encounters may be frustrated by the traditions and organizational frameworks in which they operate. The volunteers with whom she comes in contact may face serious limitations in their efforts because of insufficient resources or encouragement from the professionals. Though aware of her problems, the lawmakers may unwisely seek remedies not tailored to the special features of cancer, leaving her unaided and fostering public disappointment and unwillingness to fund new expenditures for cancer. Rather than personal, this woman's problems are intensely social. They represent manifestations of systemic shortcomings of health care in the United States when applied to modern health problems.

## "MODERN" DISEASE AND THE
## ORGANIZATION OF HEALTH CARE

In part, the hypothetical patient's problems are "social" because the popular misconceptions about cancer aggravate the emotional problems that necessarily accompany the disease. More fundamentally, though, her difficulties are social in nature since they arise from an incapacity of the present health care system to reliably handle the major health problems of modern society. The present U.S. health care system is the legacy of an earlier historical era. Today, a "modern" variety of disease whose characteristics contrast significantly with those most prevalent in years past now dominates the health concerns of Americans. Unfortunately, the characteristics of the health care system inherited from the past render it unable to effectively meet the needs of actual and potential victims of diseases identifiable as characteristic of modern times. Because cancer is only one of many modern diseases, the difficulties that the health care system encounters in controlling its effects are applicable to many health problems in advanced industrial society. Since cancer is perhaps the most prominent and problematical of the modern diseases, its successful control may provide the key to planning a more effective general organization of health resources.

Modern diseases—those that cause the most widespread fear and mortality in contemporary society—are distinctly different from those that produced terror and death in earlier generations. Most obviously, diseases like coronary thrombosis and cancer are not infectious. Among causes of death, the twentieth century has witnessed a decline in infectious disease accompanied by an increase in ailments not readily transmitted from person to person. Three of the ten leading causes of death in 1900 (tuberculosis, influenza-pneumonia, and diphtheria) were directly infectious, while three others (gastroenteritis, chronic nephritis, and diseases of early infancy) were closely related to infectious processes.[15] By 1970, only influenza remained among the ten leading causes of death. The remaining major killers—heart disease, cancer, strokes, diabetes, cirrhosis of the liver, and arteriosclerosis[16]—are modern diseases.

Modern diseases do not occur in epidemics. Although some writers have referred to epidemics of heart disease, cancer, and even emotional disturbances,[17] they have stretched the definition considerably. Past generations experienced massive waves of illness and a visible, immediate threat of death widely distributed within the exposed population. Life-threatening modern ailments pose calculable but nonimmediate threats to specific age groups, occupations, and gender categories. Residents of cities ravaged by cholera in 1832 or influenza in 1917 experienced extreme dread for brief periods of time. Today's middle-aged men and women with histories of cancer and heart attacks in their ancestries undergo levels of anxiety that are small but continuous. The grandparents of today's adults could often minimize their exposure to contagious diseases through obvious measures. But contemporary Americans—exposed to numerous, esoteric, and often contradictory theories about the causes of cancer and heart disease—can only guess about proper precautions.

The other distinguishing feature of modern disease is its chronic nature. Although chronic disease may threaten its victim's life, it often requires several years to reach the terminal stage. The prevalence of chronic disease is directly related to the rarity of life-threatening infectious illnesses. Of course, many chronic conditions are degenerative forms of illness that accompany the aging process. The control of infectious diseases, particularly those of infancy and early childhood, has produced a population more of whose members usually live long enough to contract a chronic illness.

Several analysts have specifically identified chronic disease as the health problem typical of modern society. They have specified a variety of patient needs associated with chronic disease that correspond closely to those outlined here in connection with modern ailments.[18] "Chronic" disease as used by these authors and "modern" disease as used here are fundamentally synonymous. One major distinction between these two phraseologies does exist, though. Not all life-threatening conditions that pose major health problems in modern society are chronic in the strict sense of the word, and several chronic diseases are infectious in origin and plagued humankind well before the beginning of the industrial era. Some major causes of death in modern society—including, for example, strokes, sudden heart attacks, and some forms of cancer—kill their victims soon after the appearance of early symptoms. These conditions can only be designated as chronic if the long-term organic conditions that lead up to acute attacks are considered part of the disease process. Furthermore, chronic diseases such as leprosy and malaria are infectious in nature and caused widespread health problems long before the advent of modern times. With the understanding that the term chronic disease has acquired a specialzed usage in medical sociology, it will be used interchangeably with the term modern disease throughout this book.

Ironically, the successes achieved by the traditional health care system have produced a prevalence of disease that this system often seems ill-equipped to handle. An important factor in the prevalence of chronic diseases is that physicians have learned to control infectious maladies that often accompany them.[19] It has long been recognized that complications like pneumonia kill many sufferers of diseases associated with old age. By sparing these disease victims from fatal secondary infections, sulfanilamide and antibiotic drugs have permitted them to survive until their principal ailment becomes terminal. Not only has modern medicine permitted individuals to reach ages at which heretofore rare diseases are common, but it has also enabled them to live for extended periods while suffering from chronic conditions. Effective control of infectious diseases that precede or accompany modern ailments has strikingly altered the pattern of fatal illness during the twentieth century. As Glazier notes, heart disease and cancer

> have increased by 268 percent and 240 percent respectively since 1900 in terms of deaths per 100,000 people. Other chronic diseases, such as general arteriosclerosis and diabetes, have emerged as leading causes of death. Of every 100 males born in the U.S. this year, 83 are likely to die eventually of chronic diseases; in 1901 the rate was 52 in 100. The likelihood of dying from an infectious disease is now about six in 100, which is about one-sixth of the rate in 1901.[20]

The spectacular success of modern medicine, which explains these figures, adds a social dimension to the problems of the modern disease sufferer—the fictional cancer patient described above, an actual cancer patient, or an individual with any chronic disease. In an important sense, the long-standing social commitment to preventing and curing infectious diseases left these patients vulnerable to modern ailments. The public health legislation and inoculation programs that have eradicated most diseases feared by past generations were entirely social in nature. They relied on the constraints of public laws and the resources of public treasuries to accomplish their purposes. Public education, often promoted by private organizations, typically aided the process of mass understanding and action against diseases like tuberculosis and poliomyelitis. Far from a problem to be resolved by individual doctors and patients, a series of social decisions made possible the conquest of infectious illness.

The vulnerability of today's population to modern illnesses exists in part because social commitments to their prevention have been relatively weak. While the United States has spent billions in search of cures for cancer and heart disease, relatively little has been commited to preventive measures directed against these ailments. Little epidemiological data, for example, have been collected to determine preventable causes of chronic conditions.[21] Although society has developed some capacity to control modern diseases and, in many cases, to prolong the lives of their victims, little has been done to prevent them on a large scale. While scientists may eventually discover remedies for more of these disorders, miracle cures on the order of antibiotics are unlikely. The net effect of social decisions to control infectious disease without preventing chronic ailments has made possible the prevalence of modern illness today. Had health and science policymakers recognized this eventuality as the control of infectious illness became close to certain—physicians had reliable weapons in their hands for the treatment of most of these ailments by the close of the 1940s—the incidence of modern diseases in the 1970s might well be lower. Social decisions and commitments, therefore, strongly affect the individual's vulnerability to modern diseases and the quality of life among persons who contract them. As Gruenberg has observed:

> . . . we must come to recognize that the socially organized application of health technology is one of the greatest epidemiological forces in the world. We have seen how the provision of medical care, while it has served as an important means of postponing death, has done so, to a great extent, by defeating the fatal complications (of chronic diseases), thus making these diseases more common in the population.[22]

And further:

> Now that we recognize that our life-saving technology of the past four decades has outstripped our health-preserving technology and that the net effect has been to worsen people's health, we must begin the search for preventable causes of the chronic illnesses (whose duration) we have been extending.[23]

Thus, the broadest questions of social policy help explain both the individual victim's condition and the technology available to treat it. Ultimately, improvement of the health of modern disease sufferers will depend upon answers to questions of this order. But much more concrete issues affect the individual patient's life in an immediate way. The way in which health professionals receive their training, the organization of medical care, and the patient's relations with health care providers determine his or her daily experiences.

Fundamentally, the U.S. health care system handles some classes of medical problems remarkably well. These include maladies that demand an intense, brief application of medical expertise such as broken bones, acute illnesses requiring surgery, and prevention and treatment of common infectious diseases.[24] Treatment for these complaints meshes well with the predominant methods governing health care delivery in our society. For any of these illnesses, the doctor relies on the patient to notice that he or she is sick and seek treatment. Both physician and patient expect a single office visit, a short series of visits, or at worst a brief hospital stay to resolve the problem. Both doctor and patient expect that an individual physician will be able to take care of the problem without another physician's assistance. The doctor would seldom refer the patient to another physician[25] and would anticipate rarely using facilities other than his or her own hospital to achieve a cure. Physician and patient alike probably expect emotional support to play a minor part in the encounter, although both frequently recognize the traditional presence of "trivial" features of medicine like the "bedside manner." Neither doctor nor patient would question the delegation of simple tasks related to treatment to a nurse or other "physician extender," but both would undoubtedly object if the extender claimed the right to make independent decisions about the procedure. Finally, the physicians have traditionally requested payment for the specific service performed, billing the patient or his or her insurance company on a "fee-for-service" basis.

The compatability of these features of health care delivery with the needs of those who suffer from modern illnesses is highly problematical. In fact, each of these features appears to neglect or contradict some important need of the chronic disease sufferer. A systematic examination of the nature of modern disease demonstrates why this class of illness requires a method of health care delivery different from the one that currently prevails.

### Detection Cannot Rely on Patient Initiative
Several key characteristics of modern disease suggest that patient initiative in the classical sense may be inadequate for bringing doctor and patient together. For acute disorders, the individual's condition generally becomes manifest in easily visible ways. A hip fracture or appendicitis presents obvious symptoms, capable of motivating the patient to seek medical attention in short order. Severe pain or disability, though troublesome, performs the vital function of encouraging the seeking of medical attention before the associated malady has progressed too far to respond to treatment.

But because of their usual chronicity, modern diseases may develop unnoticed by the victim over a period of years or even decades. Many American males who experience unexpected heart attacks, for example, may become noticeably ill only after cholesterol has accumulated in their circulatory system for years. It appears that significant mortality from myocardial infarction might be prevented by physicians who realize the risk of heart disease in older American males, making conscientious efforts to advise patients of the risk, and treat conditions that typically precede heart attacks (e.g., angina) whenever possible. Because the potential victims of arteriosclerosis may themselves notice few alarming symptoms, the physican incurs primary responsibility in preventing premature death or long periods of pain, anxiety, and disability.

Greater initiative by the health care provider is particularly necessary in reducing mortality from cancer. While critics note that early detection is not without its problems, a glance at five-year survival rates for the most frequent varieties of cancer provides evidence for the value of early detection. In general, the cancer patient's chance for survival is 30 percent greater if his or her illness is treated while still localized than if it has spread to the surrounding region.[26]

Yet half of the types of cancer most frequently afflicting Americans remain undetected until they are widely diffused.[27] Several distinct phenomena seem likely to have combined to produce this discouraging statistic. Many cancers, first, may produce no symptoms detectable to the victim before they spread far beyond the site at which they originate. Second, many individuals may neglect the symptoms they do detect either because they are apathetic about illness or fearful of learning the causes of their abnormality. Both these factors, which make patient initiative an unreliable way of detecting cancer early, are equally important among those who suffer from other chronic diseases.

The characteristics of modern illnesses, therefore, demand a more interventionist approach to healing than the health care system now provides. It is premature at this point to make specific recommendations about which part of the system should incur primary responsibility for assuming the initiative in detecting chronic disease. But several specific types of activity appear necessary. First, the system should identify individuals whose occupation, way of life, or genetic background predisposes them to ailments like heart disease, cancer, diabetes, and strokes. Second, health professionals must devise methods of effectively detecting early signs of disease. Finally, health care providers must formulate concrete methods of alerting individuals to their risk, motivating them to seek early detection and preventive treatment, and changing their behavior to reduce the likelihood of morbidity.

Numerous dilemmas are bound to arise in this enterprise, even if it becomes a widely accepted objective of public policy. Increased activism by a health care agency, for example, could encounter serious opposition from those concerned with maintaining privacy in the doctor-patient relationship. Collection of data on the genetic backgrounds, occupations, and life-styles of individuals to determine levels of risk bears an alarming resemblance to widely criticized surveillance of private citizens by government and business. But present reliance on the initiative of individuals—occasionally garnished with publicity campaigns stressing the importance of early detection and dangers related to smoking and lack of exercise—is inadequate. The health care system will have to create mechanisms that, in effect, extend the physician's authority outside the confines of his or her office to heighten awareness and promote prompt action among the public.

### Treatment Cannot Be Episodic

The characteristics of modern illnesses make them unsuitable for discontinuous treatment, either in a doctor's office or hospital. Once again, current treatment of these illnesses tends to emphasize control rather than cure. Victims of heat attacks and strokes must live with the possibility of renewed crises. Cancer patients, even those who have undergone apparently successful surgery or other therapy, continuously face the possibility that their malignancy will recur. Chronic conditions typically necessitate continuing care of several kinds, including follow-up therapy (such as administration of anti-hypertensives in heart cases and hormone or chemotherapy following cancer treatment), monitoring the effects of long-term drug maintenance, and watching for signs indicating the presence or approach of new or recurrent sysmptoms. Patients typically require many return trips to the doctor and often several readmissions to hospitals.

In many ways, the present-day health care system is far from ideally suited for this purpose. The physician working on a fee-for-service basis as a solo practitioner or on a "quota" system at a health maintenance organization tends to have an episodic orientation to illness. Rapid, single method cures are much more gratifying "products" for both patient and physician than maintenance in a continuing though tolerable state of illness. Wishing for a final cure, the patient dislikes the long-term regimens and changes in his or her way of life that chronic illness often demands. Perferring the satisfaction of a clear-cut medical success and the convenience of charging a single fee for a single visit, the doctor looks unhappily at the prospect of treating the same case again and again, a process that may be accompanied by complications in bookkeeping and billing for either a solo or group practice.

Just as individual physicians have reasons for avoiding commitments to continuing care, so do hospitals. Studies have shown that hospitals tend to make the highest profits during the early days of a patient's stay, during which time the patient utilizes services such as diagnostic testing, surgical preparation, and operating room support.[28] The chronically ill patient would use fewer of these services per day of hospitalization than the patient admitted for an acute condition or elective treatment. In terms of their traditional offerings, hospitals typically find it more profitable to treat illness in an episodic manner. In an effort to explain the inadequacies of the general hospital in treating chronic illness, Terris specifies a broad range of services that these facilities often lack. He writes:

> the changing character of disease—the emergence of chronic diseases as the most important causes of illness, disability and death—has exposed the inadequacies of the general hospital. No longer can such a hospital stand alone; it must provide the central core of a complete health care center, one which comprises facilities for ambulatory care, inpatient care for both acute and chronic illness, day care, rehabilitation, and skilled nursing home care, as well as outreach services for public health nursing and organized home care. Such a center is not an ideal but a necessity; without it we shall continue to provide fragmentary, uncoordinated, and inadequate care, and we shall continue to clog the general hospitals for the care of acute illness with patients who do not need their expensive services but have no place to go because other types of facilities and services are not available.[29]

## Treatment Requires More Than One Doctor

The characteristics of modern diseases make it difficult or impossible for a single physician working in isolation to treat them in the most effective way possible. The most obvious feature requiring cooperation among physicians is that modern disease sufferers often require treatment by individuals in several different specialties. An internist in community practice, for example, may be the first to treat a patient who has suffered a heart attack. The internist may at some point determine that the patient would benefit from the care of a cardiologist. The cardiologist may, in turn, determine that coronary artery bypass surgery is indicated and refer the patient to an individual specialized in these procedures. After the operation, the surgeon will quite likely return the case to a cardiologist (though not necessarily the same one) to "manage" the case—monitor the patient's condition, prescribe drugs, and so on—until he or she has recovered from surgery. Modern diseases are complex, affecting many organ systems simultaneously and spawning secondary ailments from time to time. Hence, they frequently require the services of physicians commanding widely divergent specialized fields of knowledge.

The technical complexities involved in cancer treatment may be greater than those found in the management of any other modern disease. A look at the methods physicians now use in dealing with Hodgkin's disease, a form of cancer that recent research efforts have made significant progress in controlling, provides an illustration of the range of technical tasks involved in modern cancer treatment. Treatment of Hodgkin's disease epitomizes the so-called multimodal form of cancer treatment, in which physicians utilize a combination of chemotherapeutic, radiological, and surgical procedures to diagnose and cure the malignancy. In determining the stage that the malignancy has reached in each patient, physicians may perform surgical procedures to take biopsies of internal organs such as the liver and remove entire organs such as the spleen. They are likely to perform radiotherapeutic procedures when the disease is in an early stage and combinations of radiotherapy and chemotherapy in later stages. Each type of procedure is itself quite complex. Physicians must decide which radiotherapeutic "fields" (specific combinations of body regions) to irradiate, at what levels of intensity, and for what duration. They must select among numerous courses of chemotherapeutic treatments on the basis of the disease stage and the patient's overall capacity to tolerate treatment. Each course of chemotherapy itself involves combinations of several drugs, each of which must be administered for a specific period of time, the entire sequences requiring repetition several times. The number of modes of treatment indicated appears to increase at later stages of the disease, and treatment procedures are especially complex in cases where the malignancy has reappeared following an earlier remission.[30] If the success physicians have experienced in treating Hodgkin's disease is an indication of the complexity on which improved management of other cancers depends, cancer treatment in the future is likely to become even more complicated and mutimodal than it is at present.

The technical complexity of cancer treatment strongly suggests that even the most competent and best informed physician would find it impossible to manage all aspects of a cancer case. The treatment procedures for Hodgkin's disease suggest that members of several medical subspecialties must participate in the management of a single patient. Determining the stage of a particular case of Hodgkin's disease, for example, may require consultation of a hemopathologist. Staging is crucially important in this type of illness because different stages indicate quite different courses of treatment. Radiation therapy will require a radiotherapist, and chemotherapy will require an oncologist or at least a specially trained internist.

Cancer patients may require the services of several different physicians for reasons only peripherally related to the technical tasks that treatment requires. Some physicians may feel comfortable treating cancer patients in early stages of the disease, but not in its later stages. As in Hodgkin's disease, the concrete tasks of treatment may be simpler in early stages. Later stages may demand palliative treatment, for which the original physician may not feel adequately prepared. But physicians may not feel comfortable treating later stages of cancer for personal reasons as well. Not every doctor feels comfortable interacting regularly with a dying human being.

Therefore, observers of cancer treatment have sufficient reason to believe that effective cancer control cannot take place unless patients receive care through the efforts of a number of physicians. This task could conceivably be accomplished by referring the patient from practitioner to practitioner, or by frequent exchange of knowledge about cancer treatment among doctors. Isolation from either of these two processes makes the physician who treats cancer considerably less effective than he or she might be. The ability of a physician practicing in isolation from other members of the profession to remain abreast of the latest developments even in his or her own field is highly problematical. Isolation of this kind may be more serious in cancer treatment than in other modern diseases. The major advances in cancer treatment in the past few years do not appear to have come in the form of "breakthroughs," which would eventually reach even the most isolated physician. Instead, they seem to be subtle in nature, consisting of small advances that may add up to additional years of useful life for the patient whose doctor is abreast and skillful in the applications of new techniques.

Unfamiliarity with medical innovation creates several problems for effective patient care. First, the physician may essentially give up treating the patient because of overestimating the intractability of the illness. Wakefield draws a convincing connection between relative isolation within the medical community, lack of current information, and excessive pessimism in the treatment of cancer. He comments:

> Not all doctors know the survival rates that are now being achieved. From the limited perspective of a private practice, the family physician—with his own personal experience pressed most sharply in his consciousness—does not get a broad perspective on the chances of dealing with specific forms of cancer. . . . (This generates) a disquieting degree of misinformation among medical men about the likely outcome of these highly manageable forms of early cancer.[31]

Among physicians who are aware of the basic advances in cancer treatment, relative isolation can still create serious problems. If the patient's life is threatened, for example, physicians are often tempted to utilize drugs and procedures whose effects they do not fully understand. The socialization of doctors emphasizes innovation, and physicians often receive their training at medical schools and hospitals that are advanced research sites. In practice, though, their innovative behavior tends to become imitative. This is most true when the practicing physician's knowledge is incomplete and the patient's life is in immediate danger. At this point, "imitative behavior tends to be substituted for comprehensive personal understanding" of an uncertain medical technique.[32] In the absence of other practitioners who may be readily consulted, even a physician with the greatest possible concern for the patient may cause unnecessary suffering. This possibility is especially strong in terminal cancer, where chemo- and radiotherapeutic techniques can cause extreme discomfort and deterioration if not used with the greatest of care and understanding.

Many factors may prevent the cancer patient from receiving the benefits that pooling of knowledge or readily made referrals among physicians may bring. These factors may be present even among physicians who are highly conscientious and well trained. The busy physician may not have sufficient time to read about new developments in medical journals, or to acquire a familiarity with the large volume of research results that are published regularly. But shortages of time and volume of knowledge are only part of the problem. The pattern of social relationships surrounding medical practice strongly affects the diffusion of knowledge and the transfer of patients from practitioner to practitioner. While journal readership may alert some physicians to new developments and to the existence of especially effective referral centers, adoption of new techniques in medicine and referral of patients are intensely social processes. As a classic study by Coleman, Katz, and Menzel points out, the most likely source of information to which a doctor will turn for information about a new drug is his or her local colleagues.[33] An important consequence of this feature of the medical community is that many physicians become isolated from sources of new information. Doctors in this position are likely to include, first, those who are out of contact with medical innovators—good examples might be older physicians and those practicing in rural areas. Second, noninnovators include physicians who are simply isolated from their colleagues, such as those who do not have fully privileged hospital affiliations or do not regularly attend hospital conferences.[34]

Similar blockages to exchange of information and patients are likely to be more serious in cancer, where treatment processes are often highly complex. In adopting techniques similar to those involved in treating Hodgkin's disease (or feeling confident about making referrals to physicians skilled in such techniques), a physician would have to ask many detailed questions about specific cases. In order to begin a treatment process or make a referral, the physician would have to feel comfortable about approaching a colleague personally and repeatedly. The traditional independence of physicians, prestige differences among them, and financial losses associated with seeking infomation or referring patients may all obstruct the cooperation among doctors necessary for optimal treatment of cancer.

### Treatment May Require More Than One Hospital

Just as the patient with a modern disease is unlikely to find a single physician willing and able to treat every aspect of the illness, he or she may find it difficult to procure all the necessary services under one roof. Once again, this problem arises from the medical complexity and multistaged progression of modern illness. As in the case of physicians' services, the clinical features of cancer may make it difficult for individual hospitals to provide all the services a patient will need during the course of the illness. And just as physicians may not feel psychologically prepared to interact with patients at all stages of their illness, hospitals may be unwilling or unable to make the commitments of resources necessary to meet all the patient's needs.

The importance of advanced technology in modern cancer treatment plays an important part in requiring cancer patients to use at least two hospitals during the course of their illness. Many features of cancer diagnosis and treatment today require the use of large, extremely expensive medical apparatus. Perhaps the best example of such technology is computerized tomography. This procedure allows physicians to "scan" internal tissues without performing exploratory surgery. Because of its ability to provide needed diagnostic information without the risks of surgery, computerized tomography has become extremely popular among cancer specialists in recent years. Both the hypothetical colon cancer patient with whom this chapter began and the patient with Hodgkin's disease would be likely candidates for computerized tomography. Despite its utility in cancer diagnosis and staging, computerized tomography devices (CT scanners) are very costly; their purchase is likely to be burdensome to the average hospital.

Like diagnosis, cancer treatment today relies heavily on large, expensive machines. Radiation therapy, for example, makes use of extremely high-voltage particle accelerators. "Megavoltage" equipment, which mechanically resembles devices used in high-energy physics research, has replaced older, less powerful radiation therapy devices using radioactive cobalt in many cancer treatment centers. The therapeutic advantages of the newer machinery appear to be considerable. Megavoltage equipment may allow physicians to avoid errors in treatment that may prove fatal to the cancer patient. By making the irradiation of wider body areas possible, megavoltage equipment reduces the possibility that radiation therapy procedures will miss regions affected by malignancies. The importance of such technical advantages—and, closely associated with these, the frequent need for cancer patients to be referred from hospital to hospital—is illustrated by the comments of a specialist in Hodgkin's disease:

> The use of small (cobalt-60) units, operating at treatment distances of 80 cm. or less, results in a patchwork quilt of small treatment fields which invite frequent technical errors. The patient with previously untreated, potentially curable Hodgkin's disease deserves optimal treatment the *first time*. When the requisite equipment and/or therapeutic expertise are not available in his community, the patient should be referred to the nearest major medical center for precision radiotherapy.[35]

The expenses associated with purchase and operation of devices such as the CT scanner and megavoltage equipment make it impossible for many hospitals to acquire them. Even if a hospital chooses to acquire equipment of this kind, it may be prevented from doing so by public regulatory agencies. Health systems agencies in many localities have taken steps to prevent hospitals from purchasing CT scanners, fearing that the machines will be underutilized and that the unnecessary costs of their purchase and financing will make medical care more expensive. Public policy issues related to the purchase of megavoltage equipment are similar to those arising from the CT scanner. Regulatory agencies appear to have reasonable grounds for limiting the deployment of heavy equipment related to cancer diagnosis and treatment. Expenditures for hardware related to the treatment of other modern diseases have often been found to be unnecessary. Investigators determined, for example, that in 1967 31 percent of the hospitals in the United States that had open heart surgery facilities had not used them for a year, and analysts point out that duplication increases costs.[36] Because costs limit the distribution of important components of cancer treatment, patients may have to seek treatment at sites less conveniently located than their community hospitals.

Perhaps the least even distribution of hospital resources occurs in the posttreatment phase of modern illness. Whether treatment is successful or not, the patient often requires specialized services after its completion. Patients who have undergone successful surgical procedures for cancer often require rehabilitation. For example, they must relearn speaking after laryngectomies; they must learn the use of prostheses following amputations. If the hospital at which the surgery was performed, though, does not have rehabilitation facilities, the patient will have to look elsewhere. Cancer patients whose conditions have proved unresponsive to therapy require specialized postoperative services as well. Often, these individuals need palliative care, consisting of administration of pain-killing drugs and emotional support. Specialized palliative care units facilitate this treatment by employing a specially trained staff and providing physical facilities designed to facilitate frequent family visits. All hospitals, however, do not have palliative care units. Some hospitals seem to send dying patients elsewhere as a matter of policy, deeming terminal patients unprofitable, lacking adequate physical facilities for their care, or encountering difficulties in assigning staff to the necessary duties. Analysts must also ask themselves whether the personal disinclination of hospital adminsitrators to systematically address the needs of dying patients also limits the availability of such services to a relatively small number of institutions.

### Treatment Must Include Emotional Support

While emotional support is a useful addition to many medical procedures, it plays a crucial part in the life of patients with persistent and life-threatening illnesses. The protracted nature of modern illnesses is conducive to despair among its victims. Unpleasant and time consuming therapy as well as recurrences of conditions believed cured tends to cause depression and, in extreme cases, may lead to suicide.[37] As indicated above, the fear of dread disease lowers the quality of life for many patients. Emotional support is a critical component of modern disease treatment at every stage of the individual's career as a patient.

As with the fictional patient described above, fear may be extremely intense during the diagnostic (pretreatment) period. While a problem for those seeking to minimize the disruptive effects of serious illness on victims' lives, anxiety has more concrete implications. Patients with extreme fear of a suspected illness may avoid conclusive diagnosis and delay treatment beyond tolerable limits.[38] Individuals who doubt the efficacy of medicine in curing the suspected illness tend to avoid both diagnosis and treatment.[39] For the patient who procrastinates long enough to render medical intervention fruitless, this doubt becomes a self-fulfilling prophecy.

The treatment stage seems to introduce two typical fears into the patient's mind: fear that medical treatment will be ineffective and fear of treatment itself. Large numbers of cancer victims doubt that physicians can help them in any material way. Equally important, patients anticipate the treatment process with great alarm. According to one important study, patients awaiting treatment for cancer may fear surgical mutilation, extended suffering and pain, financial devastation, the suffering of dependents, and abandonment by a repelled spouse.[40] Unfortunately, the anxiety associated with the treatment of serious illness does not seem to be reduced by knowledge about the treatment process and familiarity with the experiences of other patients. Again in the study of cancer, a national survey of 3,000 respondents indicates that personal acquaintance with a cancer victim is more important in producing fear of the disease than any other factor.[41]

The need for emotional support in the posttreatment stage is obvious. For the patient recovering from surgery, emotional support may make the difference between a successful recovery and a ruined life. Patients recovering from kidney transplants and colostomies need understanding and encouragement from those around them to adjust to fundamental changes in body processes. Women who have undergone mastectomies and hysterectomies often need assistance in overcoming threats to their gender identity. In addition, patients whose treatment has been essentially palliative, only temporarily successful, or unsuccessful need assistance in adjusting to oncoming death.

In addition to the threat that unresolved anxieties related to longlasting and life-threatening illnesses present to the patient on the emotional level, disturbed emotional states may harm the therapeutic process. Fear of the treatment process may motivate the patient to abandon orthodox medical care and seek out treatment by quacks.[42] Doubt about the efficacy of treatment may induce the patient to disobey medical recommendations and perhaps avoid the threatment process entirely.[43]

Despite the need for health care providers to take the patient's emotional needs seriously, many features of medical care delivery reduce the patient's chances of receiving the required services. Perhaps the most important reason is that administrators of hospitals and clinics often regard emotional support services as "exotic" accessories to the treatment process. Emotional support provided either by specialized personnel in one-to-one contact with the patient or in group settings may not be covered under existing insurance arrangements. Administrators may not consider such services easily "marketable" to patients or their families, since they are not as concretely or obviously necessary as more traditional aspects of medical care. Finally, physicians may harbor orientations that limit their ability to consistently or effectively provide emotional support to cancer patients. They may simply lack sufficient time to provide this complex and demanding service. In addition, their professional socialization may provide neither the skills nor concern required.

## THE NEED FOR CHANGE

To recapitulate, a health care system capable of ameliorating the threat of cancer in modern society must perform the following functions on a continuous and reliable basis: initiation of treatment aided by health professionals, continuity of care from one episode of illness to another, sharing of knowledge and patients among physicians, making a wide variety of hospital services conveniently available to each cancer patient, and providing cancer patients with emotional support when necessary. The general pattern of relationships among health professionals and hospitals appears to severely limit the capacity of the present system to perform these functions. Even without addressing the crucial issue of cancer *prevention*, health professionals, institutions, and the public face the necessity of making difficult changes in the manner by which Americans receive health care if cancer control is to be more than a disappointing slogan.

The health care system must undergo two types of changes in order to improve its capacity to control cancer. First, local professionals and organizations must become better able to perform several important functions on their own. It is reasonable to expect community practitioners to maintain as high a level of knowledge as possible about cancer detection and treatment, to include concerns for emotional needs of cancer patients in local medical practice or hospital settings, and to locate equipment necessary for early detection of cancer in places conveniently reached by residents of every community. Second, and of perhaps greater ultimate importance, health care providers must coordinate services available only at selected geographical locations. If medical hardware such as CT scanners and megavoltage radiotherapy equipment can be economically deployed in only limited numbers, their availability to patients everywhere must somehow be assured. If physicians in subspecialties too minutely defined to be widely distributed are needed to help cancer sufferers widely dispersed over a large geographical region, some mechanism must be instituted to bring doctor and patient together. Thus, the system must both improve the cancer-related services performed in each community treatment setting and enhance the coordination of activities taking place at many distant sites to accomplish the goals of the National Cancer Act.

As suggested throughout this chapter, many basic features of the social relations surrounding health care in the United States severely restrict the capacity of the system to perform these functions. Several well-known analysts of the health care system have characterized the present health care system as a loose collection of uncoordinated units highly unsuited to the control of modern disease. Glazier, for example, identifies the still predominant fee-for-service payment system as a manifestation of the fragmentation of the U.S. health care system. Fee-for-service payment, he writes, is a feature of medical care inherited from the era of contagious disease, when the most important illnesses could be most effectively treated as single episodes. When applied to modern illnesses, though, this form of payment merely accentuates the attempt of the system to regard chronic disease—whose treatment requires long-term management and coordination from one patient visit to the next—as episodic.[44] In a comprehensive overview of the present system's organizational features, Hyman illustrates the fragmented quality of such episodic treatment by noting that patients are often forced to utilize several different hospitals whose quality is not always consistent and whose services are not necessarily coordinated.[45] Although American physicians appear to be abandoning the traditional solo practice for group practices of one kind or another,[46] their immediate objective seems to be the sharing of office expenses and reducing their hours worked. Group practice will not contribute to the spread of knowledge if all physicians involved have similar specialties and educational backgrounds. If these features of health care in the contemporary United States are unsuited to the control of the modern disease in general, they are especially unsuited to the control of cancer.

It is tempting to look to regional health planning as a means of augmenting the health care system's capacity to control cancer. Initiated and administered by a central agency, a regional plan could help coordinate the divergent professional roles required for effective detection and reliable, continuing treatment of cancer. They could promote the exchange of knowledge among health professionals that would make the care they provided both more appropriate and economical. As suggested in other contexts, regional plans to coordinate hospitals could

> create a coordinated hospital system in each region which successively links together the small peripheral hospitals, the medium-sized district hospitals, and the large teaching hospital centers to create a two-way flow of patients and personnel. This would include the organization of all patients requiring more complex services, and of personnel requiring further training, who would move from the periphery to the center, and an organized program of clinical consultation, education, and other assistance by specialized personnel who would move from the center to the periphery.[47]

In fact, the cancer control provisions of the National Cancer Act are an attempt to restructure health care—or, at least, health care in one specific and highly important area—along these lines. These provisions emphasize the importance of coordinative efforts on the regional level. They directly address the needs of cancer patients by encouraging outreach and early detection, promoting the exchange of knowledge among professional personnel and referral of patients from periphery to center, and aiding the development of continuing and comprehensive care.

But highly similar legislative mandates in the past have encountered serious difficulties in achieving their goals. After all, the concept of regional health planning is hardly new. The Hill-Burton Hospital Construction Act of 1946, for example, contained provisions for linking "base, district, and peripheral" hospitals into regional systems, and it failed to produce significant results in this area.[48] Although numerous legislators and planners appreciate the importance of the social technology represented by regional coordination of health care, adoption of the technology has been considerably slower than the physical technology of modern medicine. By providing a detailed picture of the attempt to apply this social technology in a specific region, this book attempts to demonstrate how existing patterns of social relations prevent the health care system from reliably meeting the cancer patient's needs, even though modern society in many cases possesses the understanding and physical technology to do so.

## NOTES

1. American Cancer Society, *1977 Cancer Facts and Figures* (New York: American Cancer Society, 1976), p. 3.

2. Richard Severo, "Cancer: More Than a Disease, for Many a Silent Stigma," *New York Times* (May 4, 1977).

3. D. Oken, "What to Tell Cancer Patients," *Journal of American Medical Association* 86 (1961): 1126.

4. F. Davis, "Uncertainty in Medical Prognosis, Clinical and Functional," in W.R. Scott and E.H. Volkart, eds., *Medical Care* (New York: John Wiley, 1966), pp. 311-321.

5. Jim McIntosh, *Communication and Awareness in a Cancer Ward* (New York: Prodist, 1977), p. 33.

6. Severo, op. cit.

7. Ibid.

8. Ibid.

9. Susan Sontag, "Disease as a Political Metaphor," *New York Review of Books* 25 (February 23, 1978), pp. 29-33. See especially p. 33.

10. Susan Sontag, "Illness as Metaphor," *New York Review of Books* 24 (January 26, 1978), pp. 10-16. See especially p. 12.

11. Susan Sontag, "Images of Illness," *New York Review of Books* 25 (February 9, 1978), pp. 22-29. See especially p. 28.

12. D. Colburn and C.R. Pope, "Socioeconomic Status and Preventive Health Care Behavior," *Journal of Health and Social Behavior* 15 (1974): 67-78.

13. Lu Ann Aday and Ronald Andersen, *Access to Medical Care* (Ann Arbor, Mich.: Health Administration Press, 1975).

14. David Mechanic, *Medical Sociology* (New York: The Free Press, 1968), p. 131.

15. W.H. Glazier, "The Task of Medicine," *Scientific American* 228 (April, 1978): 13-17.

16. American Cancer Society, op. cit., p. 14.

17. Ibid., p. 14.

18. E.M. Gerson and A.L. Strauss, "Time for Living: Problems in Chronic Illness Care," *Social Policy* 6 (December 1975): 12-18.

19. E.M. Gruenberg, "The Failures of Success," *Health and Society* (The Milbank Memorial Fund Quarterly) 55 (Winter, 1977): 3-24.

20. Glazier, op. cit., p. 14.

21. Gruenberg, op. cit., p. 21.

22. Ibid., p. 20.

23. Ibid., p. 22.

24. A. Wildavsky, "Doing Better and Feeling Worse: The Political Pathology of Health Policy," *Daedalus* 106 (Winter, 1977): 106-1125.

25. S. Shortell and O.W. Anderson "The Physician Referral Process: A Theoretical Perspective," *Health Services Research* 39 (1971): 86-94.

26. D.C. Miller, "What is Early Detection Doing?" *Cancer* 37 (1976): 426-432. See especially p. 428.

27. Miller, op. cit., p. 428.

28. J. Wood, "Operating Revenue," in W. Cleverly, ed., *Financial Management of Health Care Facilities* (Germantown, Md.: Aspen Systems Press, 1976).

29. M. Terris, "The Need for a National Health Program," *Bulletin of New York Academic Medicine* 18 (January, 1972): 24-31. See especially pp. 28-29.

30. H.S. Kaplan and S.A. Rosenberg, "The Management of Hodgkin's Disease," *Cancer* 36 (1975): 796-803. Article provides comprehensive summary of Hodgkin's disease treatment modalities.

31. J. Wakefield, "The Social Context of Cancer," in R.J.C. Harris, ed., *What We Know about Cancer* (New York: St. Martin's Press, 1970), p. 216.

32. K.E. Warner, "Treatment Decision Making in Catastrophic Illness," *Medical Care* 15 (January, 1977): 19-33. See especially p. 22.

33. J.C. Coleman, E. Katz, and H. Menzel, *Medical Innovation* (Indianapolis: Bobbs-Merrill, 1966), p. 62.

34. Ibid., p. 82.

35. Kaplan and Rosenberg, op. cit., p. 4.

36. Herbert H. Hyman, *Health Planning* (Germantown, Md.: Aspen Systems Press, 1976), p. 43.

37. William A. Nolen, *The Making of a Surgeon* (New York: Random House, 1968). Chapter 13 contains a sensitive discussion of the emotional aspects of chronic disease. See especially pp. 152 and 153.

38. B. Kutner and G. Gordon, "Seeking Care for Cancer," *Journal of Health and Human Behavior* 2 (Fall, 1961): 171-178.

39. R.M. Battistella, "Factors Associated with Delay in the Initiation of Physicians' Care among Late Adulthood Persons," *American Journal of Public Health* 61 (July, 1971): 1348.

40. B. Cobb et al., "Patient Responsible Delay in the Treatment of Cancer," *Journal of Health and Social Behavior* 15 (1954): 67-78.

41. G.M. Levine, "Anxiety about Illness: Psychological and Social Bases," *Journal of Health and Human Behavior* 3 (1962): 30-42.

42. Cobb et al., op. cit.

43. Battistella, op. cit.

44. Glazier, op. cit., p. 16.

45. Hyman, op. cit., p. 45.

46. J. Bryant et al., *Community Hospital and Primary Care* (Cambridge, Mass.: Ballinger Publishing Co., 1976), pp. 33-34.

47. Terris, op. cit., p. 28.

48. Ibid.

# Chapter 3

# The Cancer Control Program and Its Service Region

According to many observers, eventual control of cancer and other modern diseases will require availability of resources not included in the traditional array of services that health professionals and organizations offer the public. The preceding chapter suggests that a health care system capable of providing these services must operate in a manner quite different from the one that enabled humankind to conquer infectious diseases. Aware of the need to institute new services and promote substantially greater cooperation among health care providers to make sure that these services were widely available, the framers of the National Cancer Act cancer control provisions reiterated the concern for regional coordination of health care. The provisions of the act reflect the necessity of establishing a new social technology for the purpose of controlling cancer, one that departs from the traditional independent functioning of health care providers. The present chapter examines the needs and resources related to cancer control in a specific geographical region. It then discusses the methods selected by a group of innovators funded under the National Cancer Act to promote adoption of the social technology needed for more effective control of cancer. By identifying serious shortcomings in the region's cancer-fighting resources, this chapter lays the groundwork for questioning whether the methods suggested by the National Cancer Act are adequate for the tasks it hopes to accomplish as well as determining which additional methods might be of greater utility.

The cancer control effort that this book examines took place under the auspices of an eminent university medical center in a large

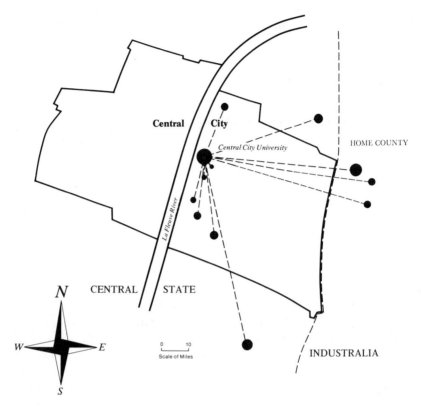

**Figure 3-1.** Central City and Vicinity Showing University Hospital and Affiliates

midwestern city. To safeguard the anonymity of the individuals and organizations that took part in this effort, the discussion will refer to the location as Central City and to the institution as Central City University. Under grants from the National Cancer Institute, faculty in many specialties at the university medical center organized the Central City University Cancer Control Program. The goals of the program ran parallel to those that the National Cancer Act had articulated. As a statement by the program's leadership to its funding agency began:

> The University . . . recognizes its responsibility to ensure rapid and effective dissemination of existing knowledge about cancer to medical practitioners and other health professionals in the community. [Through our specialized cancer control program] we propose to translate promising

research findings into practice, with the long-range goal of reducing cancer incidence, morbidity, and mortality.

The university-based cancer control program attempted to pursue these aims with the aid of eleven other hospitals in the Central City region. Several of the methods that the program later adopted amounted to serious attempts to promote regional coordination among previously isolated professionals and organizations. Within this framework, the program's major efforts aimed at inducing the region's providers of cancer-related services to transcend their traditional limitations and concerns.

As Figure 3-1 shows, the cancer control program concentrated its efforts in a region encompassing the east side of Central City and Home County in the neighboring state of Industralia. Like Central City, Home County and Industralia are fictional names for real places. The region depicted in Figure 3-1 includes a wide variety of people and land usages. Its urbanized parts, serving as home for persons of nearly every class, race, and ethnic background, in many ways typify the modern American metropolis. The satellite municipalities surrounding the major urban center and the semirural parts of the region experience many of the health-related problems of nonmetropolitan areas in the contemporary United States. Because this region encompasses so complete a cross-section of modern American life, the problems facing its health care providers and the omissions in the services they provide appear likely to reflect issues related to cancer control throughout the United States.

## THE SERVICE REGION

Located at the vortex of a megalopolis that stretches several hundred miles along the La Fleuve River, the Central City metropolitan area encompasses a vast mosaic of subregions, districts, and neighborhoods, whose boundaries are depicted in Figures 3-2 and 3-3. The region as a whole contains one of the highest concentrations of heavy industry in the United States, with major industrial areas located on Central City's east side and in Home County, Industralia. Referring to Figure 3-2, Districts 9 and 10 both contain areas of light manufacturing, including electrical appliances and machine tools among the most important. The river front section of District 9 contains an important warehousing industry associated with shipping and receiving manufactured goods as well as a narrow strip of retail businesses and professional offices along the river. The eastern part of District 10 and adjoining sections of Home County are heavily in-

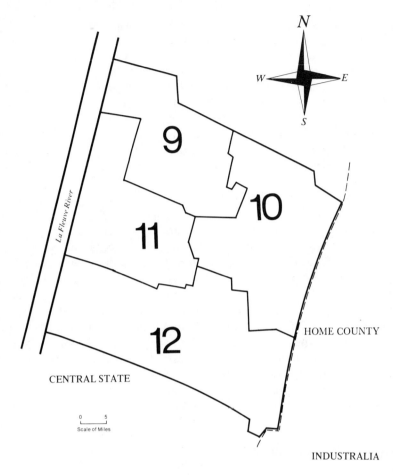

**Figure 3-2.** Central City's East Side Showing District 11

dustrial with large complexes of steel manufactuiring, oil refining, and petrochemical production dominating the economic and physical landscape. The southern part of District 10 contains a wide variety of working- and middle-class housing. Many successful black families occupy desirable, well-maintained, single-family dwellings in the central part of the district. White middle-class families predominate in the extreme southern part of the district. District 12, particularly its eastern half, tends to house upper middle-class whites. Districts 9 and 11 represent the characteristics of the so-called inner city. Both areas house largely black residents and present the observer with a general impression of decay. Owners of the districts' characteristic

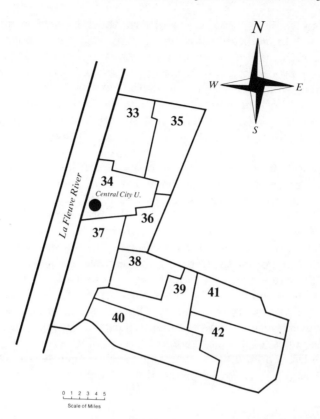

**Figure 3-3.** District 11 Showing Neighborhood Areas and Census Tracts

three-story walk-up residences typically avoid making repairs, a policy that building inspectors condone, perhaps out of simple necessity. Unemployment is a perennial problem in both districts, indicated by the large number of idle men visible on major streets during the warm months. With the exception of the warehouses and light industrial plants in District 9, few major sources of employment are available to the community for the uneducated population. Retail businesses outside the river front area operate under a continual threat of robbery, and they have become scarcer and scarcer over the years. Deserved or not, large parts of both Districts 9 and 11 have a reputation for being dangerous places to visit or traverse.

Perhaps the region's most striking contrasts in residential patterns and land use occur in Home County. The northernmost third of Home County is occupied by heavy industry, the middle third by working-class housing including numerous black and Mexican-

American families, and the southern third by upper middle-class residences. In addition, this large county contains much farmland and a few forested areas near which vacation homes have been built. A traveler proceeding southward through the county would begin in a massive, smoke-enveloped industrial complex, encounter row on row of tract housing ranging from dilapidated to new as he continued south, and find spacious dwellings surrounded by large lots at the end. In addition, the traveler would pass through several semirural pockets during the course of the journey.

Table 3–1 provides a statistical overview of the districts composing the service region of the cancer control program. The residents of District 12, an area that strongly resembles the typical American suburb although it is situated within the boundaries of Central City, generally enjoy the highest incomes in the service region of the program. The home of many professionals and business managers, District 12 also boasts the region's highest average level of education. The high percentage of residents aged below fifteen years and low proportion of individuals over sixty-four reflect the character of the district as a dormitory community whose qualities are more conducive to rearing children than retirement. District 10, an area containing many sources of industrial employment and stable working- and middle-class communities, has the second highest average income in the region. The lower proportion of children under fifteen and

Table 3–1. Selected Demographic Characteristics of Cancer Control Program Service Region by District, 1970[a]

| Demographic Characteristics | Districts | | | | Home County |
|---|---|---|---|---|---|
| | 9 | 10 | 11 | 12 | |
| Total Population (Thousands) | 942 | 958 | 352 | 548 | 480 |
| Age (Percent) | | | | | |
| Under 15 | 33 | 29 | 27 | 32 | 32 |
| 15 to 64 | 58 | 63 | 64 | 61 | 61 |
| Over 64 | 9 | 9 | 9 | 6 | 7 |
| Average Income (Thousands of Dollars) | 8.1 | 13.0 | 10.0 | 13.2 | 11.5 |
| Average Years of Education | 10.55 | 11.58 | 11.57 | 12.07 | 11.76 |

[a]Data in this table were assembled from a variety of sources, including Health Systems Agency data, census tracts, and local planning studies.

higher representation of adults over sixty-four suggest that District 10 serves as home for people in every stage of the life cycle. Home County, with its great variety of social strata and land use, falls between Districts 10 and 12 in age distribution, though its residents receive lower average incomes than either of these districts. The figures in Table 3-1 reflect the inner-city nature of Districts 9 and 11. These two districts have the lowest average income in the region and, taken together, the lowest average educational level. The high percentage of children under fifteen suggests a high birthrate; the large population wedged into the region's second smallest district indicates serious crowding. While Districts 9 and 11 are alike in many respects, District 11 does better on the average in both income and education. Because of the presence of Central City University in District 11, its population is somewhat older, and living conditions are apparently less congested than in District 9.

Much variation in racial composition, land use, and living conditions is visible even among the neighborhoods that compose District 11. A short-lived regional health planning effort during the early 1970s provides several graphic illustrations of this variation. The District 11 study had two objectives: first, to collect demographic and epidemiological data in order to determine the region's health needs, and second, to formulate proposals for comprehensive health planning in the area. Figure 3-3 illustrates the location of the neighborhoods in District 11, University Heights, the area in which Central City University is located, is one of ten neighborhoods composing District 11.

The most obvious distinction between University Heights and other District 11 neighborhoods is in racial composition. As Table 3-2 indicates, University Heights is one of only two District 11 neighborhoods with a majority of white residents. The only neighborhood in the area with a greater percentage of white residents is South Haven, a long-standing ethnic community, many of whose residents hold jobs in railroad yards nearby. Residential segregation is indeed striking in District 11, with half the neighborhoods more than 90 percent black. The pattern is sadly reminiscent of countless other inner-city areas throughout the United States. Perhaps differently from other urban core areas, though, District 11 neighborhoods no longer seem to be in the process of racial transition. A comparison of the percentages of black residents in 1960 and 1970 reveals major changes in few neighborhoods. Apparently, the changes that transformed the area had already run their course by the 1960 census. Areas to the south of District 11, however, experienced marked changes during the 1960s. Three neighborhoods immediately south

Table 3-2. Percentage of Black Residents in District 11 Neighborhoods, 1960 and 1970

| | | Black Residents | |
|---|---|---|---|
| | | 1960 | 1970 |
| Community Areas[a] | | (Percent) | |
| Elmdale | (33) | 83.9 | 78.9 |
| University Heights | (34) | 37.1 | 31.1 |
| Market Square | (35) | 99.3 | 99.3 |
| Fillmore | (36) | 99.1 | 99.1 |
| Riverwood | (37) | 89.1 | 95.8 |
| Davis | (38) | 91.8 | 87.3 |
| Germantown | (39) | 98.3 | 98.9 |
| Fairfield | (40) | 96.0 | 96.9 |
| South Meadows | (41) | 76.7 | 85.4 |
| South Haven | (42) | 31.4 | 31.2 |

[a]Figure 3-2 illustrates the location of community areas, the numbers associated with each appearing on the map.
Source: U.S. Census, 1960 and 1970.

of Riverwood, for example, became predominantly black during that decade, one neighborhood going from 63.8 to 97.5 percent black, another from 9.0 to 69.0 percent, and the third from essentially zero to 82.7 percent. Important demographic changes of a different nature continue to occur, however. That is, nearly every neighborhood area in District 11 lost population between 1960 and 1970 as substandard housing was razed and little high-density redevelopment took place (see Table 3-3).

The diversity visible within the cancer control program service region suggests that the problems related to risk of illness and access to resources are complex. In an important sense, the task of the program is to help provide and arrange cancer-fighting resources in a manner tailored to the complex needs of *this specific region.* Stated in terms of resources, the problem of constructing such a system is threefold. First, effective detection and treatment require availability of very specific resources. Second, cancer control on a regionwide basis requires arrangement of these resources in a manner that allows each component (personnel, equipment, and organizations) to contribute to the effectiveness of every other component. Finally, all components of the system must be accessible to the entire population at risk. The discussion now turns to an examination of the

Table 3-3. Population Changes in District 11 Neighborhoods, 1960 to 1970

| Community Areas | | Percent Change |
|---|---|---|
| Elmdale | (33) | −35.2 |
| University Heights | (34) | −26.4 |
| Market Square | (35) | 0.1 |
| Fillmore | (36) | 5.3 |
| Riverwood | (37) | −33.8 |
| Davis | (38) | −8.8 |
| Germantown | (39) | −24.7 |
| Fairfield | (40) | −39.5 |
| South Meadows | (41) | −15.3 |
| South Haven | (42) | −15.3 |

Source: U.S. Census, 1960 and 1970.

supply and arrangement of existing resources to help specify the actual changes that the cancer control program would have to make to achieve its goals.

## AVAILABLE RESOURCES I: THE SUPPLY

As outlined in Chapter 2, reducing the morbidity, mortality, and psychological trauma associated with cancer requires the existence of a specific set of resources. Two resources discussed in this chapter are necessary for control of serious diseases of all kinds. These include hospital and physician services, resources that can be enumerated at least initially in a straightforward fashion. Chapter 2 suggests that other resources are particularly important in controlling modern disease. These include high technology equipment, early detection, and emotional support, the adequacy of which in a given region may be more difficult to evaluate. While not covering an exhaustive list of the resources necessary for cancer control, a look at the supply of resources in these five areas begins to provide a picture of the gaps between existing and optimal cancer control in the cancer control program service region.

### Hospital Beds

Table 3-4 provides data on resources basic to the control of all diseases in the region. According to the table, the cancer control program service region contains 7,745 hospital beds for a population of 3.28 million. Within the region, there are 2.32 hospital beds for

Table 3-4.   Medical Resources Available in Region by District, 1970[a]

| Medical Resource | Districts | | | | Home County |
|---|---|---|---|---|---|
| | 9 | 10 | 11 | 12 | |
| Physicians per 1,000 Population | 1.63 | 0.71 | 0.95 | 0.49 | 1.1 |
| Hospitals | 20 | 10 | 7 | 4 | 5 |
| Hospital Beds: | | | | | |
| Long-term | 34 | 24 | 9 | 19 | 19 |
| Short-term | 2,127 | 1,743 | 678 | 1,445 | 1,647 |
| Total Hospital Beds per 1,000 Population | 2.29 | 1.84 | 1.95 | 2.52 | 3.47 |
| Number of Miles Traveled to Hospital | 2.9 | 4.8 | 4.6 | 4.0 | 3.9 |

[a]For source of data, see Table 3-1 (ff.).

every thousand residents, the ratio ranging from 1.84 in District 10 to 3.47 in Home County. Limited bed space may sometimes present residents of the cancer control program service region with barriers to hospital admission. No district within Central City approaches the national average of 3.5 hospital beds per thousand residents; only Home County equals this ratio of hospital beds to population. Neither Home County nor any Central City district approximates the 4.5 beds per thousand limit of the Hill-Burton Act. Hospital beds per thousand decrease with proximity to the inner city, the lowest ratios occurring in Districts 9, 10, and 11, and the highest ratios visible in District 12 and Home County. The lowest ratio observed in the region occurred in South Haven, where there were 1.7 beds for every thousand people.

But, despite the seemingly low ratios observable in this region, it is difficult to conclude that the area suffers from a major shortage of hospital beds. Only one of the twelve hospitals associated with the program reports an occupancy rate of 100 percent. The average occupancy rate among the twelve hospitals was approximately 80 percent, with the least fully utilized hospital reporting an occupancy rate of 70 percent. If availability of hospital beds within the region as a whole is considered an adequate indication, no compelling evidence emerges to suggest that this is a major problem.

## Physicians and Physicians' Services

While observers of the cancer control program service region can argue on the basis of occupancy rates that the area contains an adequate number of hospital beds, physicians and physicians' services present a different picture. Table 3-4 provides convincing evidence that the area as a whole suffers from a shortage of doctors. With the possible exception of District 9, the ratios of physicians to population presented in Table 3-4 are well below those of Central City and the United States. While there were 1.9 physicians for every thousand Americans in 1970,[1] and 1.9 for every thousand residents of Central City, the cancer control program service region contained only 0.95 physicians per thousand people. This region had exactly half the city average. Some parts of the area seemed especially undersupplied. District 12, for example, an area still in a period of rapid growth, had the lowest district average. Older population centers seemed to fare better in this respect, with District 9, accessible from the central business district on the west side, enjoying the highest ratio of doctors to population in the region. Depressed inner-city areas, though, appeared to suffer the worst undersupply. Within District 11, for example, the ratio of physicians to thousand residents varied from around 1.5 in University Heights and adjacent parts of nearby neighborhoods, to zero—no physician practices—in Market Square, Germantown, and Fairfield.

Lack of adequate physician services is best indicated by the widespread use of hospital emergency rooms for nonemergency care. Care from these sources has many drawbacks, including hurried delivery by busy practitioners, episodic treatment of ailments that require conscientious follow-up, and long waits for attention. Nevertheless, resort to emergency room treatment among the poor is frequent in some parts of the program service region. In 1970, for example, the District 11 study reported that over half the patients at hospital emergency rooms in the area did not have emergent illnesses.

## High Technology Equipment

Again, optimal management of cancer cases often depends on the availability of recently developed high technology equipment. Accurate diagnosis of cancer may be aided by CT scanning or the use of ultrasound devices, equipment that detects masses via sound wave resonance. As in Hodgkin's disease, megavoltage equipment is often required to give patients the best chance of recovery. Several hospitals in the program service region possess high technology equipment of this kind. According to data furnished by local health systems agencies, eight hospitals in the region possess whole body CT scanners, while ten hospitals offer radiation therapy utilizing mega-voltage equipment.

Determining whether this equipment represents an adequate supply requires a measure of guesswork. The question of how many pieces of high technology equipment represent an adequate supply for a given region is highly controversial among health planners, hospital administrators, and physicians. The controversy over the number of CT scanners that a region requires is especially heated and well publicized.[2] Following the above discussion of the supply of hospital beds, though, it seems reasonable to interpret an under-utilization of existing equipment as an indication that the region possesses an adequate number of devices, if not an oversupply. The American Cancer Society, for example, provided researchers with utilization data on three hospitals within the region that possessed linear accelerators, a widely used megavoltage device. None of these hospitals utilized the equipment to full capacity, with actual utiliza-tion rates varying between 36 and 70 percent. Hospitals within the region tended to report similar utilization rates for other high tech-nology equipment. Among a selection of hospitals within the service region, none reported 100 percent utilization of their ultrasound equipment, with the utilization rate varying between 30 and 80 percent of capacity. According to the utilization criterion estab-lished then, the region evinced no shortage of megavoltage equip-ment or ultrasound apparatus. Unfortunately, neither the local health systems agencies nor the American Cancer Society could supply data on the utilization of whole body CT scanners. Utilization patterns for other high technology equipment, however, suggest that CT devices should be adequately available.

### Early Detection Facilities

Although no central agency in the Central City area could provide complete data on early detection facilities, the importance of these resources makes at least an estimate of their availability indispens-able. For this purpose, researchers associated with the program made several limited but conscientious attempts to determine what re-sources were available for residents of the region who sought diag-nostic services for the early detection of cancer. These research efforts included: (1) a series of items in the Professional Community Survey to determine the early detection facilities available at hospi-tals associated with the cancer control program, (2) a separate survey of all public and private agencies in the region that seemed interested in early detection of cancer, and (3) a spot check of several private health providers in the region.

According to these surveys, several sources of early cancer detection examinations were available to residents of the program service region. Of the twelve hospitals covered in the Professional Community Survey—one was the Central City University Medical Center, the eleven others were hospitals associated with it in the cancer control effort—half offered cancer-screening services, typically as part of their outpatient department activities. Of forty public and private agencies contacted—researchers using mailed questionnaires and telephone follow-up succeeded in contacting about 70 percent of a sample of fifty-six organizations—seven reported that they provided cancer screening or detection services such as chest X-rays, Pap smears, and breast examinations. Prominent among those agencies provideding cancer screening were the Central City Board of Health and the Metropolitan Screening Clinic, a private facility. Both the board of health and the Metropolitan Screening Clinic provided multiphasic screening utilizing batteries of automated tests and physician examinations. The board of health offered these services at five community health centers scattered throughout Central City, three of which were located in the program service region. The Metropolitan Screening Clinic, located on the city's west side, was outside the region but still reasonably accessible to its residents via public transportation. Both organizations provided services similar to well-known cancer detection facilities like the Strang Clinic in New York and the Fox Chase Cancer Center in Philadelphia. Other agencies that provided cancer detection services included community action organizations and religious groups. The spot check of four private health providers indicated that one did offer screening services to its regular patients.

Residents of the program service region, thus, did have places in their vicinity to go if they desired cancer screening. But availability of this important service is less reliable than it appears at first glance. First, the individual desiring screening must have a fairly sophisticated acquaintance with the health care resources of the area in order to locate a screening facility. Usually, the regular sources to which most area residents turn for health care do not offer this service. Second, the screening activities of many of the providers surveyed were either limited in scope, in early stages of their development, or experimental. Several of the public and private agenices, for example, screened for only a single type of cancer such as cancer of the breast or cervix. While the Central City Board of Health planned to screen over 25,000 individuals per year at its community health centers, it had succeeded in annually processing less than 40 percent of this total when this research was conducted. Expansion of its activities, the agency noted, depended on the receipt of federal grants. The Metropolitan Screening Clinic, whose scope of activities and volume of patients the board of health hoped to emulate, charged $80 per visit at the time of this survey, a price too high for many of the individuals in the region. Finally, operators of screening activities generally reported a follow-up problem. Too often, individuals whose examination revealed suspicious symptoms failed to procure conclusive diagnosis and treatment. Noting that this problem was particularly severe among poor people, the board of health did not include tests in its procedure for which they felt follow-up would be particularly unlikely.

Interest in early detection appeared to be growing among both consumers and providers of health care in the program service region at the time of this research. But several indicators suggest that existing services are inadequate. First, the task of locating an early detection facility appeared to require a measure of sophistication not universally found among those who might seek early detection. Second, and perhaps more important, publicly supported early detection facilities seemed to possess too little capacity to handle the demand for their services. Observers reported long waiting lists of applicants for screening services at board of health facilities. By the criterion applied to hospital beds and high technology equipment, the degree to which existing capacity is utilized, the cancer control program service region appears to be undersupplied with early detection facilities.

### Emotional Support

Of all the resources needed to control cancer and its effects on human beings, the services least accessible to convenient observation are related to emotional support. For this reason, judgments of whether regions possess adequate supplies of these resources must remain guarded. Emotional support has always been part of medical care, and the most important activities in this area may take place spontaneously between cancer patients, their personal intimates, and the professionals who care for them.

Services specifically identified as emotional support for those affected by cancer in the program service region include the following programs and personnel:

1. A "death and dying" nurse at the university medical center. This

nurseing role is specifically designed to aid emotional adjustment among terminal cancer patients. Although the individual occupying this role also takes care of the patient's physical needs, by no means an undemanding duty, the nurse has special interest and preparation for counseling dying patients. At least one other death and dying nurse practices in the Central City area (though not within the cancer control program service region), and others are receiving training necessary to perform the function, usually combined with more traditional nursing roles.

2. Community support services. Although many community and religious organizations provide support for the seriously ill and dying, the American Cancer Society stands out as the leader in the field. A program known as "Cancer Call-Pac" in the Central City area invites any individual affected by cancer—an individual afflicted with the disease, a person who suspects he or she has a malignancy, or a relative of a cancer victim—to call for help at any hour of the day or night. Volunteer staffs who answer these calls are composed of cancer survivors, members of families affected by cancer, and pastoral counselors. These individuals provide emotional support, or refer the caller to others who can provide more specialized help. In addition, the American Cancer Society provides support services to individuals who have undergone specific types of cancer treatment. "Ostomy clubs," groups of individuals who have undergone colostomies, provide an opportunity for individuals who have undergone these operations to express their anxieties and share experiences with others who have gone through the procedure and adjusted to the changes it has necessitated. A similar program called "Reach to Recovery" aims at aiding the adjustment of women who have undergone mastectomies. Both the ostomy programs and Reach to Recovery begin by sending volunteers to visit patients at the hospital. Ostomy patients are then invited to participate in semitherapeutic group meetings.

3. Informally organized activity. Several groups whose members wish to assist each other in adjusting to cancer-related problems have appeared from time to time in the Central City area. Most of these seem to consist of those close to cancer patients rather than patients themselves. One group, for example, consisted of women whose husbands had recently died of cancer; another formed somewhat later, of parents of children with cancer. These groups reflect the strenuous nature of emotional proximity to the cancer victim. Not only do these individuals face personal sadness and anxiety, but also confusion about what they can and should do, what their relation to health care professionals should be, and how

they can avoid becoming a burden to the patient and health care provider.

Although many health professionals and lay people in the Central City area are concerned with the problem of emotional support and make efforts to provide appropriate services, many indications suggest that these needs remain unmet. Officials of the American Cancer Society, for example, state that insufficient support is available for the relatives of cancer patients. Individuals who have sought emotional counseling have also noted difficulties. They report great problems and extended search periods before being able to locate the professional or group with the interest and skill they need. Several patients and relatives of patients contacted during the study, in fact, indicated that they started their own groups because they were unable to find existing groups that met their needs. Initiative of this kind speaks well of the individual. But the necessity of such initiative speaks poorly of the health care system offering emotional aid to those affected by cancer.

Several important features of the atmosphere surrounding more concrete aspects of health care for cancer patients suggest that organized efforts to provide emotional support encounter serious barriers. One professional with extensive experience in long-term health care, for example, reported that hospital administrators were reluctant to commit resources to such activities, noting that their informal and unquantifiable features made them difficult to incorporate into the ongoing functioning of hospitals and did not lend themselves to convenient billing procedures. According to a representative of the American Cancer Society, this administrative attitude has prevented hospitals from instituting permanent education and emotional support programs for cancer patients, although they might allow short-term, demonstration activities to take place on their premises. In addition, resistance from physicians was noted, practitioners not wishing patients to discuss alternative medical techniques and compare experiences with Reach to Recovery and Ostomy Club volunteers. In sum, emotional support services in the Central City region are available, but typically seem incomplete, difficult to locate, and poorly institutionalized in organizations providing conventional health care.

As the National Cancer Act suggests, the goals of cancer control require concrete, "brick and mortar" facilities, professional personnel, and a variety of "supporting services" that are not always part of the health care system's traditional offerings. In the program service region, shortages seem least serious in the concrete areas (including hospital beds and high technology equipment) and most serious in the professional services area and "support" functions such as early detection and assistance in emotional adjustment for patients. The gaps between humankind's present understanding of cancer and the actual ability of health care providers to aid cancer victims and their families, though, become clearest in an examination of interrelations among components of the health care system and the special combinations of needs expressed by individuals in the cancer control program service region.

## AVAILABLE RESOURCES II: THE SYSTEM

Given the special needs of cancer patients, an investigation of the tasks facing any regional effort to control the disease must begin with a look at the available supply of each needed resource. But the most important problems in cancer control become obvious only in an investigation of the public's access to these resources. The availability of unused capacity at a CT scanning site, for example, would do the patient little good if the physician were unable or unwilling to refer the patient there. While the general question of access to health care has received much attention from health services researchers,[3] access is a much more complex issue for cancer management than most other diseases. For the cancer patient, simple access to a physician is not enough. The principal issue is, instead, one of access to *appropriate* care, providing the patient with the variety of medical, hospital, and high technology services required to treat each facet of the illness. Determination of whether appropriate care of this nature is available in a given region requires a more detailed investigation of existing services, taking into account the specific offerings of health care professionals and organizations and the distribution of these resources over the area encompassed by the region.

It would be a gross error, for example, to interpret the relatively high ratio of physicians to the population in Dictrict 9 as an indication that district residents enjoy access to appropriate care for cancer or any other disease. The services many of the physicians located in District 9 provide are often neither accessible to district residents nor appropriate to their needs. The vast majority (74 percent) of District 9 physicians are specialists and have offices located along an incongruously affluent river front strip of the district. These physicians base their practices not on the needs of older, poor, and minority residents of District 9, but on clientele referred from physicians all over the region. The section of District 9 where the offices of these specialists are concentrated is easily accessible from the west side central business district and attracts patients from that area. The same is likely to be true of many of the physicians in District 11. Because a significant proportion of these doctors are highly specialized faculty members of the university medical center, their skills and interests are often more appropriate to the needs of a widespread regional population than local district residents.

The orientation of large numbers of District 9 and 11 physicians to highly specialized and regional practices leaves residents with a limited selection of primary care practitioners. Although primary care is usually associated with diseases that do not threaten life, it is a critical component of any regional system that aims at controlling cancer. Primary care physicians are, in a manner of speaking, the best "instruments" of early detection, and they typically play the key role in referring patients to sources of more specialized care. Whatever resources a region might possess, they do not fully benefit individuals with cancer unless these patients procure care from a physician able to determine their needs, refer them to other practitioners when necessary, and admit them to hospitals with the particular service facilities they need.

Recalling the significance in cancer of continuity from treatment episode to treatment episode and a high degree of coordination among participating physicians, the services available to many inner-city residents appear inadequate. The District 11 study reports, for example, that the entire district contains several specialized health facilities (infant welfare stations, mental health centers, and venereal disease facilities) but only one community health center and a small number of community physician practices. The study observations on these facilities strikingly illustrate the gap between conditions that prevail in the inner-city areas of the program service region and those necessary for successful regional cancer control:

> None of these facilities offers a comprehensive range of services and most are overcrowded, understaffed, and unrelated in any meaningful way to other health institutions or community health organizations in the region. A patient requiring service must locate the appropriate doctor or clinic by trial and error, and will often wait several weeks before he can be seen by a doctor or appropriate health care professional. If the patient requires an extensive amount or a wide variety of services, he may be required to visit several clinics or offices, waiting several weeks between each visit and traveling as much as forty miles in the process. Should a patient require hospitalization, he may discover that the facility or doctor has no affiliation with any of the area hospitals and that he must register as a *new* patient at a hospital emergency room or outpatient clinic!

While problems of this nature would often be less serious for residents of Districts 9 and 11 who utilized the university medical center facilities for primary care, access to this facility has not always been unproblematical. This issue will receive detailed attention later in the text.

Lack of access to important resources related to cancer is not confined to poor and minority residents in inner-city areas. While inner-city residents may face problems in obtaining the services of primary care physicians, those who live in the more affluent outlying areas and suburbs may encounter difficulties procuring specialized services. Physicians with specialized practices tend to locate in the inner city. While 74 and 78 percent of the physicians in Districts 9 and 11 classify themselves as specialists, 70 and 64 percent of the practitioners in District 12 and Home County do so.

Of perhaps greater importance, high technology equipment is more likely to be located in hospitals close to the inner city than at suburban sites. The 1975 edition of the American Hospital Association's *Guide to the Health Care Field* provides an index of the technological level at which hospitals in given areas function.[4] The 1975 edition of the *Guide* classified hospitals that provided thirty or more special diagnostic and therapeutic modalities (including intensive cardiac care units, open heart surgery facilities, X-ray, cobalt, radium, and radioisotope facilities, organ banks, premature nursery, and burn units) as high technology facilities. In the Central City region, fifteen hospitals fell into the high technology category. Of these fifteen, ten were located in the inner zone of the city, one in the city's outer zone, and four in the suburbs. Consistent with this pattern of resource location, four of the eight whole body CT scanners in the program service region are found in District 9.

While the pattern in which health professionals and equipment are located in the program service region appears to create difficulties for access to appropriate services, the factor of spatial distance compounds the problem for many of the area's residents. Inner-city dwellers and residents of outlying areas face surprisingly similiar problems in this respect. According to Table 3-4, residents in District 9 have the least distance to travel to the hospital where they usually receive services; outside the central city core, Home County residents live closest to their hospitals. But number of miles is a deceptive index of physical access. Home County residents, for example, have almost no public transportation except to and from Central City. Although individuals who live in urbanized parts of the county are indeed close to the hospitals at which they seek treatment, those in outlying areas are often quite distant. Residents in one urbanized part of Home County, for example, travel an average of only one mile to their hospitals; those living in one of the semirural, outlying areas, travel an average of 14.5 miles.

Inner-city dwellers may face serious problems reaching a hospital despite their apparent physical proximity. A glance at the services available to residents of District 11, for instance, reveals an absence of swift, direct public transportation to hospitals. This district is served by several forms of public transportation: the city bus system, a city-operated, elevated transit line, and a privately owned railroad running along the river front. Of eighteen city bus routes, only eight approach (stop within six blocks) any two of the eight hospitals in the district. Thus, few district residents enjoy direct connections between home and hospital. Likewise, the elevated transit and private railroad lines approach only two of the district's hospitals. Commenting on the inadequancy of public transportation to and from inner-city health care facilities, the District 11 study noted:

> For a person in good health who seeks a check-up or for a person with only a minor illness, trying to get to an area hospital by public transportation presents a problem in strategy and timing which wears at his patience and disrupts his day. For a person afflicted with a sudden onset of illness or hurt seriously in an accident, the worst way to get to a hospital, short of walking, would be to wait at a (city) bus stop.

For the patient with a serious though nonemergency medical problem, this lack of physical access may be equally difficult. Individuals seeking medical attention for suspected or confirmed malignancies would have to resort to public transportation if they lacked sufficient funds to procure private services or strong enough social ties to call on others for help. Older patients and individuals in pain or under the influence of debilitating medication face hardships in walking from home to public conveyances, climbing stairs to train stations, standing on crowded buses, and waiting on street corners in inclement weather.

In general, the cancer control program efforts must overcome shortages of some facilities that are crucial for the regional detection and treatment of cancer. These include physicians' services (particularly primary care in the inner city), early detection facilities, and emotional support programs. But additional problems may be identified even with resources that appear to be in adequate supply, such as hospital beds and high technology equipment. Elderly and sick individuals may find transportation to hospitals difficult to obtain, a factor that may deter them from receiving regular medical treatments or regularly visiting relatives hospitalized for cancer. The hospital to which a cancer patient is admitted may not possess the equipment or personnel necessary to give him or her the best chance of recovery, and the admitting physician may lack the necessary ties within the physician community to refer this patient to an appropriate physician or hospital. Some individuals with treatable cancers may never receive appropriate treatment because of inability to obtain primary care or to maneuver through the maze of disconnected health care facilities located in the region. The spatial and social arrangements that govern the availability of cancer-related resources, then, essentially bar large numbers of individuals from lifesaving services. Cancer researchers may well have improved cancer-fighting technology in recent years, but important features of the health care system prevent society from obtaining the full benefits of these techniques. Perhaps the best illustration of the mismatch between system characteristics and human needs is provided by a brief examination of the social epidemiology of cancer.

## RISK OF CANCER IN CENTRAL CITY: THE SOCIAL CORRELATES OF ILLNESS AND DEATH

Like most illnesses, cancer occurs with different frequencies among differing segments of the population. It has been well documented that, like most diseases, cancer incidence and mortality occur most frequently among groups with lower socioeconomic status[5] and that both illness and death from cancer occur more frequently among blacks than whites.[6] Given these facts, it is far from surprising that two heavily black and economically disadvantaged neighborhoods within District 11, Market Square and Fillmore, have cancer mortality rates approximately 40 percent higher than the district and national averages (see Table 3-5). While all neighborhoods in District 11 except South Haven and University Heights are predominantly black, the remaining black neighborhoods have lower mortality rates for a simple reason, that is, among black neighborhoods, only Market Square and Fillmore have significant proportions of residents sixty-five years of age and older. Among neighborhoods in District 11, the combination of predominance of blacks and a sufficient percentage of older residents corresponds to a very high mortality rate from cancer.

National statistics suggest an explanation for the high cancer mortality rates in District 11 neighborhoods housing high percentages of blacks in susceptible age brackets. As Table 3-6 shows, black males are about 15 percent more likely to contract cancer than white

Table 3-5. Mortality from Cancer in District 11 and United States, 1974[a] (per 100,000 Population)

| Community Area | | Deaths per 100,000 |
|---|---|---|
| Elmdale | (33) | 151 |
| University Heights | (34) | 140 |
| Market Square | (35) | 245 |
| Fillmore | (36) | 235 |
| Riverwood | (37) | 156 |
| Davis | (38) | 112 |
| Germantown | (39) | 119 |
| Fairfield | (40) | 131 |
| South Meadows | (41) | 151 |
| South Haven | (42) | 111 |
| District 11 (total) | | 172 |
| United States, 1971 | | 171 |

[a] *1977 Cancer Facts and Figures,* American Cancer Society, 1977.

Table 3-6. Incidence Rates (Age-Adjusted) per 100,000 by Site, Race, and Sex for Most Common Cancers

| Site | Rates per 100,000 Population | | | |
|---|---|---|---|---|
| | Male | | Female | |
| | White | Black | White | Black |
| All Sites | 342.5 | 397.1 | 270.4 | 256.6 |
| Breast | 0.7 | 1.0 | 75.0 | 57.6 |
| Lung, Bronchus, and Trachea | 70.7 | 89.9 | 14.4 | 14.4 |
| Prostate | 57.7 | 94.9 | — | — |
| Uterus Cervix | — | — | 14.9 | 33.6 |
| Corpus | — | — | 21.0 | 12.1 |
| Pancreas | 12.2 | 17.1 | 7.3 | 9.8 |
| Bladder | 23.5 | 12.2 | 6.2 | 4.3 |
| Colon | 33.4 | 28.2 | 29.4 | 27.8 |
| Lymphomes, all | 13.0 | 7.6 | 10.5 | 6.0 |

Source: U.S. Department of Health, Education, and Welfare, National Cancer Institute, *Third National Cancer Survey: Incidence Data,* NCI Monograph 41, March 1975.

males. Black males contract three of the most common cancers that afflict American—respiratory (including lung, bronchus, and trachea), prostate, and pancreatic—more frequently than white males. Most other cancers represented in Table 3-6 occur more frequently among black than white males as well. While prostate cancer is highly treatable, victims of other cancers more common among black than white males have low survival rates (see Table 3-7). The elevated probability of death from cancer among black males, therefore, stems in part from their greater risk of contracting particularly dangerous malignancies. The picture appears somewhat different among females. Table 3-6 indicates that white women contract cancer more frequently than blacks. Only with cancer of the cervix do black women face a higher risk. Table 3-7 suggests that even among individuals whose cancers have been detected early, blacks face a higher risk of death than whites. For most forms of cancer, the percentage difference in survival rates between whites and blacks is similar among populations with malignancies at all stages and those among whom cancers were detected while still localized.

Epidemiologists have proposed many possible explanations for the higher risk of cancer among blacks. Theories have focused, for

Table 3-7.  Five-Year Relative Survival Rates, by Stage, Race, Sex, and Site, 1955-1964

| | All Stages | | | | Localized | | | |
| | White | | Black | | White | | Black | |
| | Male | Female | Male | Female | Male | Female | Male | Female |
|---|---|---|---|---|---|---|---|---|
| All Sites | 31 | 47 | 21 | 37 | 59 | 74 | 49 | 69 |
| Breast | — | 62 | — | 47 | — | 84 | — | 77 |
| Lung and Bronchus | 8 | 11 | 6 | 6 | 27 | 40 | 23 | 26 |
| Prostate | 51 | — | 41 | — | 64 | — | 58 | — |
| Uterus | | | | | | | | |
| Cervix | — | 60 | — | 51 | — | 79 | — | 78 |
| Corpus | — | 72 | — | 40 | — | 83 | — | 63 |
| Pancreas | 1 | 2 | 1 | 3 | 4 | 5 | 3 | 8 |
| Bladder | 56 | 56 | 29 | 27 | 68 | 71 | 46 | 48 |
| Colon | 43 | 48 | 33 | 38 | 70 | 75 | 61 | 69 |
| Hodgkin's Disease | 36 | 44 | 23 | 33 | | | | |

Source: *Cancer Rates and Risks*, 2nd ed., DHEW (NIH) Publication No. 75-691, 1974.

example, on genetic factors. Others have pointed to environmental, occupational, and life-style variables that expose blacks to carcinogens. These observers note that many occupations filled by blacks involve particularly great exposure to industrial carcinogens and that cigarette smoking has increased more rapidly among blacks than whites since 1930. These facts, they suspect, may account for a 50 percent increase in cancer mortality among black men observed between 1950 and 1967, a period that witnessed only a 20 percent increase among white males.[7] Many other biological, economic, and environmental variables may account for the elevated rate of cancer deaths among blacks.

But an equally strong hypothesis is that blacks and other categories of disadvantaged individuals simply do not receive appropriate care for malignancies as often as those in the society's economic mainstream. The significantly higher than average cancer death rates observed in Fillmore and Market Square may stem in part from the fact that few physicians practice there, and the physicians who do provide services for residents of these neighborhoods maintain few strong ties to outstanding cancer specialists or major referral hospitals with high technology equipment. Table 3-7 supports this hypothesis. Suggesting that for most forms of cancer early detection alone cannot reduce the difference between black and white mortality rates, this table implies that even blacks who have their cancers caught early receive less effective treatment than whites. The hypothesis that inferior medical care helps create inequality in black and white cancer survival rates is, of course, beyond the scope of this book. But the possibility that even part of this difference may be explained by lack of access to appropriate medical services among the socially disadvantaged illustrates the mismatch between allocation of health resources and social needs. At least in the cancer control program service region, the individuals who face the highest risk of contracting cancer appear to have the poorest access to appropriate medical services.

## THE CANCER CONTROL
## PROGRAM STRATEGY

The goals of Central City University's Cancer Control Program appear well fitted with the needs of the region that it serves. A key feature that prevents the area's residents from receiving appropriate care for malignancies, for example, appears to have been lack of integration within the local health care system. Even residents who procured primary care, for example, were not assured of receiving the latest treatments available, the benefits of the most advanced high technology equipment, or the services of hospitals with specific cancer-related offerings. Perhaps the principal response of the program to this situation was an effort to establish more active relationships from the center to the periphery within the region's professional community. The cancer control program envisaged a definite "metabolic interchange" between physicians at the university medical center and local community hospitals. Under the auspices of the cancer control program, individual departments at the university medical center such as surgery and oncology formulated contractual agreements with several community hospitals. These agreements constituted the framework for an educational outreach program, through which the center hoped "to ensure the rapid and effective transfer of technology in cancer to the health practitioners in the region." In return, the contracts obliged the community hospitals to pay part of the program cost.

Actual transfer of knowledge from the center to periphery took place in two principal ways. The first method consisted of regular appearances by university physicians at the departmental conferences and so-called tumor board meetings of the community hospitals. Departmental conferences are regular meetings organized along specialty lines that constitute a regular part of hospital-based medical practice. At these conferences, physicians present clinical descriptions of cases that include data on the illness, the type of treatment employed, and the outcome of the therapy. Tumor boards are interdisciplinary groupings of practitioners specifically interested in cancer. Tumor board meetings concentrate specifically on cancer cases and are open to all interested parties.

Organizers of the community outreach program hoped that participation by university faculty would make in-hospital conferences of this kind more effective. It was expected, of course, that their presence would improve the breadth and content of case discussions. But perhaps more important, proponents of the program hoped the academic visitors would draw more physicians to the meetings. Although an active schedule of meetings is sometimes necessary for hospital accreditation, physicians often avoid them, perhaps signing attendance sheets and leaving soon thereafter. Organizers hoped that the presence of distinguished academic physicians at the conferences would increase their prestige and thus attract the attention of hospital staff more consistently.

Equally important in the educational outreach program was the opportunity for physicians at participating community hospitals to consult with university physicians whenever the need arose. Under the contractual agreements, physicians in the community hospitals were encouraged to telephone doctors at the University Medical Center for information on difficult or unusual cases. Like the visits of university faculty to medical conferences in local hospitals, the consultation program was designed to alleviate the isolation of the community physicians from sources of assistance and knowledge.

While the university medical center received financial support for the program from participating community hospitals, it placed considerably higher value on a different return on the effort it invested: increased patient referral. The center organizers considered the relation between extending opportunities for consultation into the community and the potential for increased referrals to the university a close one indeed. In an important statement of goals, the center emphasized the objective of "developing educational programs that will simultaneously result in ongoing professional education and more appropriate referrals between the medical center and community hospitals." After three years of operation, center spokesmen reported with pride that "referrals to the University Medical Center for specialized tests and treatment" had, in fact, increased.

While the tumor board program and offer of consulting services aimed primarily at improving regional integration of the physician community, a second set of programs strove to improve the quality and scope of cancer nursing services. Again educational in nature, these efforts spoke directly to unmet needs of cancer patients for diagnosis, treatment, and emotional support. According to an official statement, the primary goal of the program in this effort was "defining and supporting an expanded role for nurses in oncology" by upgrading the nurse's level of knowledge. The program efforts in nurse education may be viewed as a means of improving the health care provider's cancer-related services by adding to its capacity in two important respects: (1) improving the hospital's ability to utilize up-to-date therapies by training nurses in their administration and (2) improving the system's capacity to provide emotional support by making the nurses more aware of patient needs in this area.

During the period 1974–1977, the cancer control program developed a core curriculum in nursing oncology. These efforts produced several courses of varying content and duration. The majority of these courses were directed at improving the knowledge of cancer among registered nurses already in practice. Specific examples included a course entitled "Current Concepts in the Management of Patients with Cancer," a program covering theories of the etiology of cancer, basic concepts of chemotherapy, radiotherapy, and multimodal therapy, as well as the psychosocial management of cancer patients. An experimental effort, the cancer control program gave this course to nurses at the university medical center, administering a pre- and posttest to determine whether the instruction increased the participants' knowledge of cancer.

At later stages of its development, the program offered several courses for which the nurses who participated could receive continuing education credit from their professional association. One such course, concerning cancers affecting children, was offered to nurses at the university medical center pediatric facility. This course lasted one day and included material on the reactions of families to cancer in children. Other programs included a series of seminars for nurses at the university medical center on major varieties of cancer and a statewide series of three-day courses on similar topics cosponsored by the state division of the American Cancer Society. Designers of these courses aimed at formulating programs that nursing educators at local community hospitals could easily adapt for use at their own institutions.

The Central City University Cancer Control Program, then, utilized two of the principal approaches recommended by planners for creating a system better able to treat modern disease. First, the educational outputs of the program were designed to provide more appropriate patient care at community facilities. Postgraduate oncology for physicians would make them more aware of the latest techniques and their proper application. Oncology education for registered nurses could allow them to provide services doctors could not provide because of time pressures or personal preferences. Second, the cancer control program hoped to encourage community physicians to refer cancer patients to the university medical center through strengthened professional ties. Program officials reasoned that if community physicians more readily referred patients to the· university, patients whose physicians lacked specialized cancer skills or access to high technology equipment could benefit from these resources.

## REGIONAL NEEDS AND PLANNING GOALS

This chapter has presented an overview of cancer-related resources in the cancer control program service region. It has identified a variety of needs that apparently remain unmet. Within the cancer control program service region, individuals in several different social categories appear to encounter serious barriers to obtaining appropriate services related to cancer. Poor and black people, for example, tend to live in areas undersupplied with physicians and to see physicians whose linkages with the rest of the health care system are weak; inner-city dwellers and those in outlying parts of Home County appear to lack adequate transportation. Individuals living close to the urban core may face problems procuring hospital beds, while those in the outer and suburban rings may encounter difficulties finding doctors with the proper specialties or hospitals with sufficiently high technical capacities. Individuals who face the highest risks of cancer seem to have the poorest access to appropriate health services. The health services available to residents of the region's poorer areas are often uncoordinated with other parts of health care system, offering only episodic care for an illness whose chronic features typically require continuous management. Persons in any social category may inadvertently select physicians who do not know the latest developments in cancer treatment or who are unable or unwilling to refer them to more knowledgeable practitioners or hospitals with appropriate facilities.

It is tempting to view the Central City University Cancer Control Program strategy as an effort to solve problems that are national in scope on the regional level. Issues considered in this chapter such as the supply and distribution of health resources, access to health care, and carcinogenesis are debated frequently among policymakers and critics nationally. Within the limits of its resources and geographical responsibilities, the cancer control program appears to have formulated a highly reasonable approach. Instead of increasing the national supply of physicians, for example, the program strove to train nurses for expanded roles. Better educated nurses could, presumably, perform many of the functions now performed by physicians, effectively expanding the supply of medical services available to actual and potential cancer victims. Studies have shown that in at least one vital area of cancer control, the screening of populations for early signs of the disease, nurses perform essentially as well as physicians.[8] Instead of attempting to produce new physicians with a more balanced set of skills, another national concern, the cancer control program aimed at improving the flow of knowledge from academic medical centers to community practitioners and facilitating the referral of patients requiring highly specialized knowledge for effective treatment back to the academic center. By fostering the development of a more highly coordinated regional system of better trained personnel, the cancer control program strove to make cancer treatment less episodic than it often is at present. The program approach is highly consistent with a health planning goal of the highest national priority: containment of costs. An alternative to duplication of facilities, coordination of services should reduce costs for the whole region. Furthermore, better trained physicians seem less likely to prescribe long sequences of ineffective treatments, a major factor in the high cost of chronic disease management.[9]

The strategy of the cancer control program, though, requires a basic change in the social technology surrounding the delivery of health care in the contemporary United States. For a more efficient application of our current understanding of cancer in the lives of actual disease victims, the habitual practices and interrelations among health care providers and patients alike must undergo transformation. Some features of medical care that must undergo revision are widespread throughout American society and date back for generations; some are peculiar to the Central City University Medical Center and the surrounding professional community. Whether existing practices are recent inventions or age-old traditions, whether local peculiarities or institutions national in scope, practitioners are not likely to abandon them at the simple request of the cancer control program or any other regional planning effort. Powerful factors within the professional community stand between existing reality and the cancer control program objectives. Chapters 4 and 5 identify and discuss the significance of these barriers to success. The difficulties discussed in these chapters do not represent an exhaustive list of problems that face regional cancer control or similar efforts at innovations in health care. But Chapters 4 and 5 well illustrate one type of problem likely to arise in any regional planning effort: the influence of valued patterns of activity in existing professional communities.

## NOTES

1. Physicians per each thousand population ratio computed on the basis of American Medical Association estimate in 1973 of 366,379 doctors in the United States (*Profile of Medical Practice*, Chicago: American Medical Association, 1974, p. 95), divided by estimated population of 200 million.

2. The following articles discuss major issues related to benefits and costs of CT scanners:

S.D. Rockoff, "The Evolving Role of Computerized Tomography in Radiation Oncology," *Cancer* 39 (1977): 694-696; H. Schwartz, "The Government Puts a Damper on Scanner Bonanza," *New York Times* (December 18, 1977); S.H. Shapiro and S.M. Wyman, "CAT Fever," *New England Journal of Medicine* 294 (1976): 954-956; D.F. Phillips and K. Lillé, "Putting the Leash on 'Cat'," *Hospitals* 50 (July 1, 1976): 45-49; R. Swartz and S. Des Harnais, "Computed Tomography: The Cost-Benefit Dilemma," *Radiology* 125 (October 1977): 251-253; H.P. Greenwald, J.M. Woodward, and D.H. Berg, "Transportation or CT

Scanners: A Theory and Method of Health Resource Allocation," forthcoming in *Health Services Research.*

3. An outstanding discussion of the literature and analysis of original data appear in Lu Ann Aday and Ronald Andersen, *Access to Medical Care* (Ann Arbor, Mich.: Health Administration Press, 1975).

4. American Hospital Association, *American Hospital Association Guide to the Health Care Field* (Chicago: American Hospital Association, 1975).

5. A.M. Lilienfeld, M.L. Levin, and I. Kessler, *Cancer in the United States* (Cambridge, Mass.: Harvard University Press, 1972), p. 105.

6. V.H. Henschke et al., "Alarming Increase in the Cancer Mortality in the U.S. Black Population, 1950-1967," *Cancer* 31 (1973): 763-769.

7. Ibid.

8. See, for example, D.G. Miller, "What Is Early Detection Doing?" *Cancer* 37 (1976): 426-432.

9. K.E. Warner, "Treatment Decision Making in Catastrophic Illness," *Medical Care* 15 (January 1977): 19-33.

# Chapter 4

# The Physician Community

Societies have often waited long years between the introduction of new technologies and their general application in everyday life. The history of medicine contains numerous examples of resistance to innovations that later proved to be of inestimable value in the prevention and treatment of disease.[1] Social innovations often encounter similar resistance. Decentralization of decisionmaking in American industry, for example, has permitted certain types of businesses to grow faster and earn larger profits than the traditional vesting of leadership in a single, centrally based executive.[2] Yet in many firms, entrenched leadership or uncritical acceptance of traditional management practices has delayed adoption of the new organizational form.[3] By discussing several important features of the social relations among health professionals in the cancer control program service region, Chapters 4 and 5 attempt to demonstrate the distance between existing social technology in health care and the social technology necessary for more effective cancer detection and treatment. Perhaps of greater importance, these chapters identify practices among health professions and within organizations providing health care that threaten to inhibit adoption of the new social technology.

Again, the widespread application of recent developments in cancer detection and treatment requires adoption of a very specific social technology by the health care system. As described in the preceding section, the central feature of this technology is the systematic sharing of knowledge and responsibilities for patient care among numerous physicians and other health professionals. The social technology that currently prevails in medical practice dates from an era when industrial and medical technology faced simpler tasks than they do today. In an epoch when acute, infectious ailments constituted the principal threats to humankind's health, the lone physician administering drugs in single applications or prosecuting straightforward public health measures could utilize existing technology effectively. At present, the complex and chronic features of cancer and other modern diseases require considerably more coordination among health care providers of both an interpersonal and interorganizational nature.

Any program of cancer control must concentrate a good part of its effort on promoting coordination of activities and exchange of information within the physician community. A vigorous community of physicians, readily exchanging techniques and cases, raises the probability that the patient's contact with the health care system will be successful. As outlined in Chapter 3, the cancer control program strove to promote the growth of such a community through an educational outreach program. By making members of its medical faculty available for conferences at community hospitals and for telephone consultation, the university sought to increase the local physician's knowledge of the latest cancer detection and treatment techniques. By making contacts between its staff physicians and doctors in the community more frequent and consequential, the university hoped to encourage referral of difficult cases to its medical facilities.

The strength of the physician community—considered as either an active exchange of knowledge among practitioners, willingness to refer patients back and forth, or a combination of the two—bears directly upon the public's access to appropriate care. *Appropriate* care, once again, is more important in many respects than simple access to health care facilities or personnel. The patient receives few benefits from visiting a physician who lacks sufficient knowledge to treat the illness. This patient receives less than optimal benefits from a practitioner who does not know the latest medical techniques and may actually incur harm from a physician whose knowledge is imperfect. Because of their frequent isolation from sources of new knowledge, community physicians—particularly those dispensing primary care—may be unable to render entirely appropriate service. On the other land, the highly specialized physician in a university hospital may lack skills of a sufficiently general nature to provide appropriate care, again resulting in less than optimal treatment. Even if the specialized, university-based physician could render primary care that was appropriate in a technical sense, such care might still be inappropriate in an economic sense. The highly specialized physician who serves as the public's first contact with the health care system uses his or her time inefficiently, performing a service a less specialized individual could do equally well, and creating a scarcity of his or her specialized capacity elsewhere in the system. Services dispensed at a university medical center, moreover, tend to be more expensive than comparable activity in a community setting because a university-based medical practice employs more technology in the form of costly tests and specialized procedures than a community practice.[4]

Inappropriate care is both more likely to occur in cancer than in other diseases and to have more serious consequences when it does occur. One outcome of imperfect updating of knowledge and techniques by local practitioners is less appropriate care for the patient in a purely technical sense. Many important features of the medical technology related to cancer are relatively new, and practical familiarity with them is restricted. Isolation of physicians from appropriate communication networks can lead to inadequate treatment of patients. As late as 1970, Matthias observed that ". . . as many as 10 percent of new (breast cancer) cases are still, by modern standards, not being adequately treated when they are first present, even allowing for the fact that there is some room for debate as to what constitutes the best form of treatment."[5] Of equal significance, insufficient knowledge of recently developed techniques of cancer therapy can produce feelings of fatalism among physicians. The restricted network of professional contacts that accompanies private practice is capable of preventing physicians from realizing the therapeutic alternatives available to them. Commenting on this process, one author notes that a "disquieting degree of misinformation (exists) among medical men about the likely outcome for . . . highly manageable forms of cancer."[6]

This chapter will approach the physician community in two ways. First, it will deal with the referral process. Patient referral is perhaps the most formal type of interaction in which most physicians regularly engage. The transmission of patients from doctor to doctor involves the potential for tangible gains and losses in status and money for both the individual making and receiving the referral. Second, the chapter examines communication patterns among physicians. Both patient referral and information exchange can take place in varying degrees of formality. Information exchange may take place as an off-the-cuff query by one individual to another in a hospital corridor, or through a contractual relationship allowing one physician to ask another for guidance. A physician may ask a colleague to see one of his or her patients *via* formal, written request or as an in formal professional courtesy. These varying levels of formality in physician interrelationships may make it difficult to clearly distinguish referral from communication. This chapter does not attempt to make a strong distinction between the two features of the medical community nor to identify differences in the way each process occurs. Rather, it attempts to demonstrate the existence of distinct categories of physicians in the cancer control program service region and to specify factors that keep physicians in some categories from exchanging information and patients with physicians in other categories. The inability of physicians in some groups to exchange information and patients with physicians in others indicates a gap between the social technology envisaged by the cancer control program and that which prevails in the program service region. The unwillingness of some physicians to exchange information and patients with others or to take the necessary steps to facilitate this process constitutes a barrier to establishment of the social technology necessary for optimal cancer control. While focusing on some features of the physician community specific to the cancer control program service region, this chapter identifies difficulties that are likely to occur in regions throughout the United States.

## REFERRAL PATTERNS
## AMONG PHYSICIANS

The manner in which physicians exchange patients is perhaps the most complex feature of the delivery of medical care. Referral relationships among medical doctors may begin in the earliest years of medical practice; for some physicians, they may predate entry into medicine, as fathers who pass their practices along to sons bequeath working relationships with their associates as well as their patients. In addition, referral is a relatively rare event in medicine. Surveys in the United States and Great Britain indicate that physicians refer only 5 in 250 patients to other physicians.[7] The referral process is influenced by an elaborate series of incentives and disincentives, complexes of prestige relationships, and historical accidents. The physician whom the patient with cancer sees first is the "gatekeeper" to the entire medical care system, the individual to whom the patient looks for proper routing to the professional who can help him or her most or the hospital with the most appropriate services and equipment. Influencing the decisions of these gatekeepers may be the most difficult of the tasks that face health planners.

Several distinct networks of physicians appear likely to coexist in any given locality. Physicians in one network generally communicate with those in another only occasionally, and many doctors may never interact with physicians outside their own network. According to Coleman et al., networks of physicians are frequently based on institutional affiliation, with physicians tending to look for discussion or advice toward others affiliated with the same hospital or who share the same office.[8] Physician networks also seem to form among individuals who perceive each other's levels of medical competence as acceptable. If a doctor develops the impression that a colleague is not performing at an acceptable level, he will not allow that colleague to work with him or his patients. As Freidson notes:

> The offender is not referred patients, or, if referral must be made, only unimportant cases are sent to him. He is not consulted about problems in his specialty or subspecialty: his advice is not sought, and he is not called in to look at an interesting or peculiar case.[9]

The penalty for unacceptable performance is exclusion from the referral and discussion network. Physicians excluded in this way, though, may establish networks of their own. Freidson explains that while physicians may not allow an offender to work with them, they will "not attempt to bar him from working with or on the patients of others."[10] Thus, several networks might exist within a region, each constituting a separate system of communication and referral occurring at specific levels of perceived ability. This is not to say that distinctions among networks are always drawn according to absolute differences in competence. Legitimate differences in criteria for mutual evaluation may exist within any medical community, giving rise to distinct networks of interrelations. Physician networks often appear to have accidental components, membership being based upon personal likes and dislikes as well as specified professional criteria.

Referral behavior within a physician network is itself a complex process. Networks often appear to be internally stratified, that is, to include practitioners who are more or less prestigious within their own circles. Each network contains an economic market feature as well, in which referring physicians face financial risks and consultants receive financial benefits. A rich commingling of potential advantages and disadvantages accompanies the physician's decision whether or not to refer a patient as well as the choice about the consultant to whom the patient should be referred. An outstanding analysis of the contingencies surrounding this process of decisionmaking by Shortell and Anderson is worth quoting at length:

> The referring physician may be rewarded by having his patient receive proper treatment for his illness; by receiving a complete and prompt report from the consulting physician as to the patient's condition and future course of therapy; by receiving the patient back from the consulting physician for continuing care, or at least knowing that the patient will return to him for the next episode of illness; by increased prestige or status within the local medical community due to referral to a higher status colleague; by having the consulting physician refer some of his patients in return . . . .

Further analysis by Shortell and Anderson implies that physicians regard referring patients to others whose status differs significantly from their own as particularly hazardous. They remark:

> The referring physician's cost may include the foregone income he would have earned had he treated the patient himself; the possible psychological cost of acknowledging to the patient his inability to treat the illness; the possibility of permanently losing the patient to the consulting physician; the risk of improper treatment by the consulting physician, reflecting on the referring physician; the "fatigue" involved in poor communication from the consulting physician as to the final disposition and treatment procedures for the patient; and the possibility of losing status within the medical community by referring to a physician of lower status or by having his work-up criticized by a physician of equal or higher status.[11]

Patterns of referral within any given region, therefore, may be divided along axes of several different kinds. The discussion to follow will consider one major division among physicians in the cancer control program service region: practice at the University Medical Center versus practice in the community. The division between university and community practice is not the only criterion for identifying networks of physicians within the program service region. Many other, more complex divisions are undoubtedly present as well. But an understanding of the difference between referral behavior among community and university physicians is particularly relevant to control of cancer and other modern diseases. Cancer control, the regional medical program, and similar proposed innovations in the organization of health care all assume that stronger relations between community medical practice and university centers are desirable and feasible. An examination of the prevailing referral patterns between community and university physicians in the cancer control program service region helps specify the task to be accomplished. Specific features of the Central City University Medical Center pose difficult problems for the establishment of stronger referral linkages. Although unique features of the university medical center pose special difficulties, these difficulties should alert planners to the possibility of similar problems everywhere.

### The University Medical Center
The Central City University Medical Center plays a pivotal role in the cancer control program plan of operation. Consistent with the notion of regionalization, the university medical center provides tertiary care—highly specialized diagnostic and therapeutic services for cancer patients, with special emphasis on particularly complex cases—and disseminates information on new techniques to the surrounding medical community. To play this role successfully, any academic medical center must attract large numbers of physicians throughout the service region to its educational programs and, in turn, attract large numbers of patient referrals from them. In any regionalization effort, the quality of the relations of the central medical facility with community physicians and hospitals will largely determine the success or failure of the plan. Because the history, commitments, and methods of operation of any central facility help determine its relationship with the regional medical community, an understanding of these features must precede examination of the attitudes and behavior of community practitioners and health care organizations.

From its earliest days, Central City University set basic biomedical research as the principal goal for its medical school and associated hospitals. Within the framework of biomedical research, the university set its sights high indeed. A founder of the university at the turn of the century outlined his expectations for the medical school in very clear terms:

I do not have in mind an institution which shall devote itself merely to the education of a man who shall be an ordinary physician, but rather an institution which shall occupy a place beside the two or three such institutions that already exist in our country, one whose aim it shall be to push forward the boundaries of medical science, one in which honor and distinction will be found for those only who make contributions to the cause of medical science, one from which announcements may be sent from time to time so potent in their meaning as to stir the whole civilized world.

The medical school later adopted unusual methods to approach these extraordinary goals. Unlike most medical schools, it was housed in the same administrative unit as the university's teaching and research in biology. Founders of the medical school conceived this organizational arrangement in order to create an "organic union" between medical studies and other academic activity. Consistent with these features, the medical school played a pioneering role in the "full-time movement" of the early twentieth century. This movement among leading medical schools of the time held that clinical professors should devote their entire time to teaching and research. As a spokesman for this movement remarked, the principal purpose of establishing full-time medical faculty positions was to allow medical faculty members to "devote their main energies and time to their hospital work and to teaching and investigating without the necessity of seeking their livelihood in a busy outside practice and without allowing such practice to become their chief professional occupation."[12]

Both the goals and methods outlined by the founders of Central City University Medical School remain in use today. Central City University's School of Medicine and its medical center are staffed entirely by full-time medical faculty who have no outside private practices. Basic biomedical research still constitutes the institution's primary goal. Physicians at the university medical center are quick to contrast the goals and methods of their institution with those of other university medical centers in the Central City area. "Research is how *we* get our kicks," remarked one professor in the department of medicine. A colleague in another department characterized the faculty of a nearby private medical school as "a loose collection of private practice physicians," and a local, publicly supported institution as "just a place that produces doctors for the state."

It would be almost impossible for a medical school anywhere to maintain as pure a commitment to research as those goals and methods imply. The Central City University Medical School is no exception. In addition to research, it performs educational functions, providing medical students, house staff members (interns and residents), and fellows with knowledge on several levels. The needs of individuals undergoing each variety of training generate differing demands on the university medical center as an organization. According to a prominent authority on medical education on the university faculty, for example, individuals in different stages of their training require different case material. Students and house staff in their early years require "bread and butter" medical cases, such as infections, pneumonia, and emergency work. Fellows require large numbers of specific disease cases, such as adrenal cancer or diabetes, a need that they share with members of the faculty. While students need the diverse and "ordinary" cases they would be likely to encounter in community practice, fellows and faculty require steady supplies of cases of a single disease in order to generate the statistics necessary for scholarly publication.

Although many faculty members, moreover, would undoubtedly like to see an exclusive commitment to research at the university medical center, basic changes in the organization's environment have made this increasingly less feasible over the years. As late as the 1950s the medical center was able to attract sufficient numbers of patients through its clinics and far-flung network of referring physicians to generate all the teaching and research cases it needed. But demographic changes on the east side of Central City during the 1960s and 1970s made the patient supply much more problematical (see Chapter 3). During this period, large numbers of residents in Districts 9 and 11 relocated to the city's suburban ring, depleting the supply of patients applying for medical services through the university clinics. While the medical center had been able to pick and choose among applicants before the 1960s, rejecting those who did not constitute interesting teaching and research cases, it was later forced to liberalize its admission standards to bolster dwindling bed utilization. The university was forced to adopt a closer orientation to direct patient service than it had traditionally held. Even so, the population bases in Districts 9 and 11 had shrunk too much to generate sufficient numbers and varieties of cases through the clinics alone. Key departments in the medical center departed further from the institution's traditional orientation by initiating an educational outreach effort similar in structure to that of the cancer control program. Directing this effort at community physicians in the immediate region, the departments of medicine and surgery were able to increase referrals significantly.

But the orientation to an audience of physicians and biomedical scientists extending well beyond the immediate region is still clearly in evidence at the medical center. Far-flung linkages with physicians at locations quite distant from the east side of Central City, for example, are indicated by the geographical origins of patients receiving cancer treatment at the University Medical Center. Table 4-1 presents a breakdown by cancer site and geographical origin of all cancer patients treated at Central City University during the year 1976. According to the table about 65 percent of the cancer cases treated at the medical center came from the cancer control program service region, including 17 percent from District 11 and 47.5 per-

Table 4-1. Geographical Origins of Cancer Patients at University Medical Center by Cancer Site[a]

| Cancer Site[b] | District 11 %[c] | District 11 N | Rest of Program's Service Region % | Rest of Program's Service Region N | Central City's West Side and Western Suburbs % | Central City's West Side and Western Suburbs N | Rest of Central City Metropolitan Area % | Rest of Central City Metropolitan Area N | Outside Central City Area % | Outside Central City Area N | Site Total % | Site Total N |
|---|---|---|---|---|---|---|---|---|---|---|---|---|
| Esophagus | 2.1 | (4) | 1.7 | (9) | .9 | (1) | 1.5 | (2) | 4.0 | (6) | 1.99 | (22) |
| Stomach | 3.2 | (6) | 3.8 | (20) | 2.7 | (3) | 2.3 | (3) | 2.0 | (3) | 3.17 | (35) |
| Large Intestine | 4.2 | (8) | 6.1 | (32) | 8.0 | (9) | 11.6 | (15) | 6.0 | (9) | 6.62 | (73) |
| Rectum | 2.6 | (5) | 2.9 | (15) | 1.8 | (2) | 1.5 | (2) | 3.3 | (5) | 2.63 | (29) |
| Pancreas, etc. | 3.2 | (6) | 2.3 | (12) | 5.3 | (6) | .8 | (1) | 5.4 | (8) | 3.00 | (33) |
| Larynx | 3.7 | (7) | 2.7 | (14) | 0 | (0) | 3.1 | (4) | 1.3 | (2) | 2.45 | (27) |
| Bronchus, Lung, etc. | 11.2 | (21) | 9.9 | (52) | 6.2 | (7) | 10.0 | (13) | 11.4 | (17) | 9.98 | (110) |
| Breast | 11.7 | (22) | 12.0 | (63) | 14.2 | (16) | 13.2 | (17) | 13.4 | (20) | 12.52 | (138) |
| Uterus | 14.8 | (28) | 13.9 | (73) | 12.5 | (14) | 7.0 | (9) | 2.0 | (3) | 11.52 | (127) |
| Ovary, etc. | 1.1 | (2) | 3.6 | (19) | 1.8 | (2) | 0 | (0) | 2.0 | (3) | 2.36 | (26) |
| Prostate | 11.7 | (22) | 4.8 | (25) | 3.6 | (4) | 2.3 | (3) | 2.0 | (3) | 5.17 | (57) |
| Malignant Melanoma | 0 | (0) | 1.0 | (5) | 5.3 | (6) | 2.3 | (3) | 2.0 | (3) | 1.54 | (17) |
| Other Skin | 3.2 | (6) | 3.1 | (16) | 8.9 | (10) | 3.1 | (4) | .7 | (1) | 3.35 | (37) |
| Brain, etc. | 1.6 | (3) | 2.7 | (14) | 4.5 | (5) | .8 | (1) | 4.0 | (6) | 2.63 | (29) |
| Endocrine Thyroid | .5 | (1) | .8 | (4) | 2.7 | (3) | 3.8 | (5) | 3.3 | (5) | 1.63 | (18) |
| Connective Soft Tissue | 2.1 | (4) | 2.9 | (15) | .9 | (1) | 1.5 | (2) | 1.3 | (2) | 2.17 | (24) |
| Reticulum Sarcoma, etc. | 1.1 | (2) | 4.3 | (23) | 6.2 | (7) | 6.2 | (8) | 10.7 | (16) | 5.08 | (56) |
| Hodgkin's Disease | 1.6 | (3) | 4.0 | (21) | 3.6 | (4) | 10.8 | (14) | 4.7 | (7) | 4.44 | (49) |
| Multiple Myeloma | 1.1 | (2) | 1.5 | (8) | 1.8 | (2) | .8 | (1) | 0 | (0) | 1.17 | (13) |
| Leukemia, etc. | 2.1 | (4) | 5.0 | (26) | .9 | (1) | 5.4 | (7) | 9.4 | (14) | 4.71 | (52) |
| Other | 17.0 | (32) | 12.7 | (58) | 8.0 | (9) | 11.6 | (15) | 10.7 | (16) | 11.8 | (130) |
| Area Total[d] | 17.0 | (188) | 47.5 | (534) | 10.2 | (112) | 11.7 | (129) | 13.4 | (149) | 100.00 | (1102) |

[a]The following sites were not included in the table due to the small number of patients treated (less than 10): salivary gland; floor of the mouth, other mouth NOS; oral mesopharynx; nasopharynx, hypopharynx, and pharynx NOS; small intestine; liver, gallbladder, biliary passages; nose, nasal cavities, middle ear and accessory sinuses; other urinary organs; giant follicular lymphoma and other forms of lymphoma and riticulosis NEC; mycosis fungoids; myelofibrosis.

[b]"Cancer sites:" Large Intestine = large intestine except rectum; Pancreas, etc. = pancreas, peritoneum, unspecified digestive organs; Bronchus, Lung, etc. = bronchus trachea, pleura, lung, mediastinum, and unspecified respiratory; Breast = breast, excluding skin; Uterus = cervix uteri, corpus uteri; female trophoblastic tumors; Ovary, etc. = ovary, fallopian tube, broad ligament, vulva, vagina, and other female genitals; Malignant Melanoma = malignant melanoma of skin; Other skir = skin except melanoma; Brain, etc. = eye, brain, and nervous system; Endocrine Thyroid = thyroid and other endocrine glands; Connective Soft Tissue = connective and other soft tissue; Reticulum Sarcoma, etc. = reticulum cell sarcoma, lymphosarcoma, and other primary malignant neoplasms of lymphoid tissue; Leukemia, etc. = leukemia, acute eryhremia, and polycythemiavera.

[c]Column percentages refer to total cases for each region including those for sites omitted from the table.

cent from the remainder of the region. The majority of these cases doubtlessly came via referral. While some individuals living in District 11 certainly arrived at the medical center on their own, using the center's outpatient facilities as their regular source of primary care, the majority were referred by local physicians to specialty clinics or to the surgical services. Individuals living outside District 11 seldom seek primary care at the university. Almost all patients with cancer from Districts 9, 10, 12, and Home County present at the medical center through referral. The remaining cancer cases treated at the university during 1976 resulted from distant referrals. About 35 percent of all cancer cases originated outside the cancer control program service region.

Table 4-1 illustrates important differences between cases received through distant referral and those originating in the cancer control program service region. While cancers originating in the vicinity of the university tend to be those with the highest incidence—which include respiratory, breast, uterine, and prostate malignancies—those referred from distant places occur with less frequency in the population. While breast, respiratory, uterine, and prostate cases together make up over 49 percent of the cancer patients originating in District 11 and 41 percent of those referred from the remainder of the program service region, patients with these cancers compose only 29 percent of those referred from outside the Central City metropolitan area. Several less frequently occurring cancers—malignancies of the endocrine system, non-Hodgkin's lymphoma (reticulum cell sarcoma and other malignancies of the lymphoid tissues), Hodgkin's disease, and leukemia—compose only 5.3 percent of the cancer patients who live in District 11. Patients with these diseases, however, compose 14.1 percent of those referred from the remainder of the program service region and 28.1 percent of those referred from outside the Central City University metropolitan area. The tendency of patients with less frequently occurring cancers to originate in areas farther from the university than those with the most frequently treated malignancies is illustrated best by the referral pattern related to non-Hodgkin's lymphoma. Patients with this set of conditions represent only about 1 percent of those from District 11 and 4.3 percent of those residing in the rest of the program service region. But they compose 10.7 percent of patients referred from outside the Central City metropolitan area. More patients with non-Hodgkin's lymphoma ($N$ = 31) are drawn from *outside* the program service region than from inside its boundaries ($N$ = 26).

Several features of the data presented in Table 4-1 are entirely consistent with the university's recently expressed objective of becoming a regional referral center. Most of the cancer cases in fact originate within the program service region. The distant referrals, though, reflect the more traditional concern of the center with medical activity beyond regional significance. If the university medical center goals were purely regional, one might suspect, the types of cancer treated would be those statistically most likely in the area. In fact, certain types of malignancies are clearly overrepresented in the mix of cancer cases at the university. These overrepresentations are quite consistent with the role of the university as a national-international referral site and center for biomedical research. Any medical center with such claims would be expected to offer services so specialized that they would require a national clientele for full utilization and would attract patients from distant localities.

This pattern of cancer treatment reflects two major but distinct goals for the university medical center as an organization. Although the goals are not contradictory in a logical sense, they indicate the possibility that university physicians may have special problems related to acceptance of and by community physicians. One would expect, for example, that many physicians at the university medical center would find it difficult to place a strong emphasis on maintaining good referral relationships with doctors in their own locality. Much significant research at the university in recent years, for example, has focused on non-Hodgkin's disease lymphomas, a type of disease overrepresented among distant referrals in Table 4-1. The medical relationships that generate referrals of patients with these ailments are not primarily local or even regional. Rather than strong, local ties, physicians interested in obtaining sufficient numbers of cases for significant research must build and maintain looser, more extensive linkages with the medical profession on a national basis. While local and regional ties may arise from personal contact at educational programs, local professional society meetings, or informal social contact, national and international contacts are generated by journal articles and appearances at national meetings as well as having a general reputation for expertise in certain areas. One physician at the medical center illustrated this difference in the case of referrals for mycosis fungoides, a malignancy that has received much attention from university researchers. He noted that a university medical center physician had presented a paper on mycosis fungoides at a conference in Texas in the early 1960s. In the late 1970s, patients were still being referred from Texas for treatment of this disease!

Both in its approach to cancer and other diseases, the medical center appears to suffer from a high degree of ambivalence. The traditional commitments of the center to basic biomedical research demand commitments of resources in highly specific directions and suggest a definite mechanism for making professional contacts and attracting patient referrals. Other commitments, whether arising from the functions generally required of medical schools, new demographic trends, or changing governmental priorities, require that resources be committed in other directions and professional ties be formed through new methods. The university medical center, then, appears at present to be an organization with several conflicting sets of goals. As the discussion to follow will show, the characteristics of these goals as well as the methods the medical center has adopted to implement them are responsible for several difficulties it has encountered in its attempt to become a regional center for cancer control.

## PATIENT REFERRAL IN THE SERVICE REGION

### Norms and Realities

In order to examine the referral process within the cancer control program service region, the Professional Community Survey included questions asking whether patient referral was an important norm in the local physician community, that is, whether respondents thought such activity was desirable and encouraged in their work environment. Other items in the survey asked whether the norm was supported in practice. Specifically, the survey asked physicians associated with the cancer control program: (1) How important they felt patient referral among doctors *at their hospitals* was within the institutions at which they practiced, and (2) how important they thought referral of patients to physicians *outside their hospitals* was at the institutions where they practiced. The doctors responding to the survey generally shared the impression that considerable amounts of time, effort, and money were spent in referring patients to the appropriate place within the hospitals at which they practiced; they gave a slightly weaker impression that their hospitals expended much effort in referring patients to other health care facilities and outside doctors (see Table 4-2). Thus, the doctors we contacted seemed to accept referring patients to the place where they could get the most appropriate care, inside or outside their own institution, as an important professional norm.

Referral norms at the university medical center differed from those at the community hospitals in one important respect. While equal percentages of doctors at both the university and community hospitals thought referrals inside their hospitals received equal em-

Table 4-2.  Percentage of Physicians Who Perceive Great Importance Attached to Referral of Cancer Patients at Their Hospitals[a]

| | Physicians at Central City University | Physicians at Community Hospitals | $\chi^2$ |
|---|---|---|---|
| Referral Within Hospital | 80.0(12) | 79.2(42) | 0.09 |
| Referral Outside Hospital | 33.3(10) | 77.4(41) | 8.44[b] |

[a]Percentages in this table have been abstracted from two fourfold tables ($df = 1$) cross-tabulating site of practice with perceived importance of referral, both within and outside hospital. Figures in parentheses represent number of physicians in each category who perceive that their hospitals attach great importance to patient referral, indicated by a great amount of effort, time, and money being spent on this activity.
[b]$p < .01$.

phasis at their respective institutions, doctors at the university perceived that significantly less emphasis was placed upon referring patients to other hospitals. This finding is hardly unexpected. There is nothing surprising in the observation that doctors at an eminent medical center should expect to find adequate consultant resources for most types of cancer under the same roof. Referrals outside the medical center would most likely include only those directing the patient back to the primary care physician or routing terminal patients to sources of long-term or palliative care, fields that the university tends to deemphasize.

The survey results, though, suggested differences between the norm of regular referral and actual referral activity. The survey asked each physician whether he or she usually referred patients with specific cancers to other physicians, and, if so, where these physicians practiced. Of the seventy-nine physicians who supplied complete answers to these questions, only thirty, or 38 percent, reported that they had usually referred any type of cancer patient during the year preceding the survey. This low figure is explained in part by the type of physician on which the survey concentrated. We selected physicians who expressed special interest in cancer. Since many of the physicians responding to the survey were cancer specialists, it is probable that many of the patients they treated had come to them on referral and did not require referral elsewhere for still more specialized care. Still, the 38 percent figure seems low for a period of one year, particularly since cancer patients often require tertiary care, involving procedures beyond the scope of even the community specialist.

When referral did take place, it was not a random process. As Table 4-3 suggests, referral to physicians at the Central City University medical facility was a more popular activity among university physicians than practitioners in the community. With few economic disincentives to making in-hourse referrals, university physicians engaged in the practice relatively often. Doctors who referred cancer patients to hospitals other than those of Central City University tended to practice at community hospitals. A total of twelve physicians reported that they had referred cancer patients both to physicians at the university hospital and elsewhere. The majority of physicians reporting such activity, however, were on the staffs of community facilities.

At first glance, Table 4-3 seems to suggest an important line of cleavage between academic and community physicians, with academic and nonacademic practitioners belonging to segregated colleague networks. But much evidence suggests that the critical axis of division implied by Table 4-3 is not one of academic versus nonacademic physicians. The majority of physicians who reported making referrals to hospitals other than the Central City University facility designated that these were other academic medical centers. As noted earlier, two other university medical centers are located in Central City. While Central City University is the only academic medical center on the east side, the west side houses two important medical schools with their associated hospital facilities. The nineteen community physicians who sent cancer patients to hospitals other than Central City University appeared to be referring to one or both

Table 4-3. Percentage of Physicians Who Refer Cancer Patients to Central City University Medical Center and Other Hospitals[a]

|  | Physicians at Central City University | Physicians at Community Hospitals | $\chi^2$ |
|---|---|---|---|
| Refer to Central City University | 44.4(8) | 19.7(12) | 3.29[b] |
| Refer to Other Hospitals | 16.7(3) | 31.1(19) | 0.82 |

[a]Percentages in this table have been abstracted from two fourfold tables ($df = 1$) cross-tabulating site of practice with referral of cancer patients within the last year to university and community hospitals. Figures in parentheses are the number of physicians in each category who indicated that they usually referred at least one type of cancer case to the university or specific community hospitals during the year preceding the survey.
[b]$p < .10$.

these so-called rival institutions. Physician networks in the cancer control program service region, then, did appear to transcend the boundaries between academic and community medicine.

The tendency of some physicians in the program service region to send patients to medical centers on the city's west side raises a crucial issue. Are patients who could receive the most appropriate care at the Central City University Medical Center in fact referred elsewhere? Despite the fact that patients living in the program service region must travel farther to reach medical centers on the west side, community physicians may consider the facilities of the west side institutions more appropriate for certain cancers than those of the university medical center. The community physicians surveyed selected Central City University as a referral site more often than any other single hospital. The university medical center may, in fact, attract its fair share of referral patients in the vicinity. The west side medical centers are widely known for their work in kidney, prostate, and endocrine cancers, malignancies in which Central City University does not specialize. But the key question of actual physician decisionmaking remains open. Do community physicians refer cancer patients to facilities other than the university medical center because they offer more appropriate patient care or because nontechnical factors have deterred them from selecting the university as a referral site despite its superior medical offerings?

### Central City University and Community Medical Practice: Traditions and Animosities

Several items of evidence seem to indicate that community physicians often hesitate to refer cancer patients to the university medical center even though they could obtain the most appropriate care there. Although this study did not evaluate the concrete suitability of the university's facilities in comparison with other referral sites, many indirect indications supported this conclusion. Community physicians seemed intimidated by the university, either because of its international stature, its relationship, both present and traditional, with physicians in the surrounding community, its economic significance in the locale, or combinations of these and similar factors. Contact with physicians (either through the Professional Community Survey or a less formal, open-ended procedure conducted over the telephone) whose hospitals participated in the cancer control program educational outreach effort provided revealing glimpses into the disincentives for referring patients to the university medical center.

In general, the physicians interviewed expressed approval of the university faculty's participation in departmental conferences and grand rounds at their hospitals. Remarks abounded, such as, "The participation of Central City University faculty has greatly increased the staff's interest in our monthly oncology conference," and "They have added much variety and authority to our discussions." Physicians expressed the feeling that educational efforts of this kind were more fruitful than other sources of new medical knowledge. They enjoyed their contact with university faculty and noted that the benefits of being able to ask questions, a benefit that was unobtainable from reading journal articles by these same individuals. The diffusion of knowledge that the university had sought to encourage had clearly met with some success. As one physician practicing at a community hospital commented:

> The oncology conferences attended by University faculty have been very effective. Spreading knowledge about chemotherapy is an example. Before the (cancer control) program began, only two people here were giving chemotherapy. Now 70 to 80 percent of the staff physicians treating cancer do. The program has been especially useful in updating the knowledge of primary care physicians, many of whom read very little.

Another physician reported that he had learned of a still unpublished chemotherapeutic technique through the oncology conference that he found very useful in his practice.

The university's attempts to draw new referral patients to its medical center also seem to have achieved some positive results. Physicians reported sending patients to the university medical center for laboratory tests that were not available at their facilities. They reported referring patients to university physicians who had outstanding success in treating certain types of cancer. The area of hematological oncology seemed to be one that drew referrals most strongly, the university enjoying a good reputation for its management of leukemia and lymphomas. Doctors whose hospital staffs included no hematologists seemed especially willing to refer leukemia and lymphoma patients to the university.

Comments of other physicians, though, indicated an undertone of hesitancy about referring patients to the university medical center. Doctors interviewed reported several concrete problems that they or their colleagues had experienced in referring patients to the university. Minor reservations included the unwillingness of patients to enter the university neighborhood, which, along with District 11 as a whole, had a reputation as an area of high crime. Similarly, physicians told interviewers that their patients shied away from the possibility of being referred to the university because the area's congestion made parking difficult, and safe, convenient public transportation was perceived as unavailable.

But community physicians expressed more substantial reasons for not referring patients to university facilities. Most frequently, they cited poor communication with the university as an inhibiting factor in making referrals. As one physician remarked:

> A communication gap exists between doctors at the university and in community hospitals. The physical distance contributes to this gap. In addition, the University Medical Center often does not feed information back to the referring physician on the treatment his patient has received or how the patient is doing. Under these conditions, the community physician completely loses out. The patient's family still turns to him to find out how their relative is doing, and he can't give them an answer. Then, what if the patient gets sick as a result of his treatment at the university? This often happens with chemotherapy. Much of the time, the patient will call his physician back in the community for help. And if the physician doen't know what medication the patient was given, he can't be very much help.

Other physicians contrasted the communication process of Central City University with that of one west side academic medical center. One respondent to the telephone interviewing reported that a west side medical center had a standardized procedure employing report forms that they used to inform referring physicians about the treatment their patients received and the progress they made, a service unavailable at Central City University on a reliable basis. Although this physician said he had been able to get the information he needed from the university when he took the trouble to make inquiries, he expressed generally negative feelings: "There's too much effort involved, too much paperwork."

A survey conducted by the university in connection with earlier efforts by the departments of medicine and surgery to increase referrals through educational outreach provides more systematic data on why many physicians feel reluctant to refer patients to the medical center. As Table 4-4 indicates, the physicians surveyed appeared generally less satisfied with the university medical center than with the alternative referral sites. The quality of care did not seem to be the major concern of referring physicians. The vast majority of respondents expressed satisfaction in this area, and they also seemed quite satisfied with the university's location, permitting

Table 4-4. Satisfaction Among Community Physicians with University Medical Center and Other Referral Sites by Issue Area

| Issue Area | Percentage Satisfied | |
| --- | --- | --- |
| | With Central City University | With Other Referral Hospitals |
| Quality of Care | 91 | 97 |
| Convenience of Location | 84 | 73 |
| Admitting Procedures | 83 | 93 |
| Patient Follow-up Reporting in Hospital | 58 | 75 |
| Patient Follow-up Reporting After Discharge | 55 | 84 |
| Referral Hospital Doctor-to-Patient Communication | 80 | 90 |
| Referral Hospital Staff-to-Patient Communication | 87 | 93 |
| Return of Patients for Continuing Care | 79 | 94 |
| Composite of Above | 77 | 87 |

easier access to many east side residents than other places their physicians might choose to refer them.

The major source of dissatisfaction with Central City University as a referral site detected in the university survey is the same as that suggested by the physicians interviewed in the telephoen survey: communication back to the referring physician. As Table 4-4 indicates, the two areas related to referral in which community physicians report the lowest levels of satisfaction with the university medical center are "patient follow-up reporting in hospital" and "patient follow-up reporting after discharge." These items represent the two most important aspects of communication between hospital and referring physician, indispensable for the community practitioner's ability to perfom effective therapy when the patient is returned to his care or to communicate with the patient's family while he is hospitalized at Central City University. Physicians responding to the university survey reported satisfaction with other referral hospitals in these two areas with considerably greater frequency.

University health planners have not been unaware of the importance of maintaining good communication with physicians who refer patients to the medical center and have taken steps to correct the difficulties illustrated in Table 4-4. In 1972, the university established a liaison office to inform referring physicians of their patients' progress. The liaison office developed a form for house physicians to complete for each case referred from outside, to be processed by the liaison office and transmitted to the referring physician. Planners of the liaison office also hoped the facility would become a central place within the sprawling medical center where information on all referred patients currently occupying one of its beds was kept. In this way, the medical center could provide all referring physicians with a single telephone number, allowing them to reach a source of information on the patients they referred without an extended search through the vast hopsital system.

But the dominant commitments of the university medical center appear to have rendered the liaison office partially effective, at best. An inquiry into the office operations seems to indicate that the commitment of the medical center to its success has been small. At the time of the present study, only two individuals shared responsibility for liaison work: an administrator with several other responsibilities and a half-time assistant. It appeared that the administrator spent most of his time in other activities, principally purchasing equipment for a new research facility. If time commitments are good indications of organizational priorities, the liaison system seems indeed to be low on the list. This impression is reinforced by the inadequate office space the liaison project has received and the reported unwillingness of house staff to prepare prompt reports for referring physicians. Community physicians continue to report that it is often difficult to obtain information on the patients they refer to the medical and surgical services and to cite this difficulty in explaining why they prefer to send their patients elsewhere.

Although receiving reports about the patients they refer to the university medical center is necessary to enable the referring physicians to effectively perform their duties to the patients and their families, this feedback of information has an equally important significance in a subjective sense. It seems certain that community physicians consider this a professional courtesy, a gesture of recognition by the university physician thanking them for their referral and acknowledging their colleagueship. For physicians, who today occupy a position of extremely high status in American society, failing to receive such validation of status must be a very disagreeable experience. Other physicians may be the only category of individuals in the position to challenge a physician's status; *university* physicians, because of their special status in the medical world, may be the only people whose acts of omission may be viewed as a snub by community physicians.

Community physicians, of course, did not explain their dissatisfaction with Central City University in the language of a social scientist. But several did indicate that dealing with the university exposed them to feelings of professional subordination. Some seemed to feel the very notion that they should occasionally refer cancer patients to Central City University implied that their abilities were inferior to those of the university physicians. As one oncologist in a community hospital commented, "Why should I refer patients to the university? I *am* a cancer specialist!" Another doctor at a community hospital sardonically questioned the university's motives for promulgating the educational outreach program, asking, "Why should I be one of Dr. Newman's (the cancer control program director) guinea pigs?"

The element of disesteem that the community physician seemed to feel from the university physician occasionally took a more concrete form. Several community physicians, for example, commented that they had difficulty getting patients back from the university after they had been referred for a specific procedure. The university survey of medical and surgical referrals detected this in a more systematic way as a reason for hesitancy in referring patients to the medical center. Again referring to Table 4-4, community physicians felt dissatisfied with the "return of patients for continuing care" following treatment at the university medical center in comparison to other referral sites. In this area, community physicians perceived an important economic dimension accompanying the threat to their status. But it would be inaccurate to think of this difficulty as purely economic for the community physician. One physician expressed the feeling—a notion that is apparently widespread among the medical profession in general—that he valued his ability to work with difficult illnesses as long as he had a chance of curing or ameliorating them but became discouraged when he could do nothing for the patient. He connected his hesitancy in referring a patient to the university medical center to the impression that "they keep him there 'til there's no more to be done. Then they send him back."

A particularly powerful deterrent to referral from community physicians seemed to be fear that the university physicians would criticize their previous treatment of the patient. One physician commented that community physicians felt they could avoid criticism by avoiding referral. Again, this source of hesitation appeared to have an economic element as well: a damaged reputation could lead to a damaged practice.

The most striking mixture of perceived status and economic threats from the university—a configuration of problems that doctors could avoid by refraining from referring patients there—came from one physician who said:

> We refer very few patients to Central City University. A very bad taste for the university prevails in the locale, because the university has triggered a great many lawsuits against community physicians. This can happen because of comments the house staff at the university Medical Center make. Doctors at the university will tell patients, "My God, what did those guys (at the community hospital) do to you?" or, "If we had seen you before, we could have helped you, but not now . . . ."

Such criticism, according to this physician, was unreasonable. He explained that cases for which referral to the university was indicated were always problem cases. The poor condition of the referred patient, he commented, was not the result of poor skills of the community physician, but the depth of the medical problem itself. The doctor cited two malpractice suits pending against community physicians that comments by house staff personnel had apparently triggered. Both cases were unrelated to cancer. One was a recurrence of a hiatus hernia following surgery and the other a delayed diagnosis of ulcerative colitis. The problem, though, seemed especially serious for cancer, where clinical complexities abound and delay in diagnosis and appropriate treatment is frequently fatal.

Again and again, conversations with both university and community physicians suggested that the dominant orientations and commitments of the medical center limited its ability to extend and solidify referral linkages with the surrounding region. The apparent disesteem in which university physicians held private practitioners weakened their ability to understand the factors that inhibited the development of improved referral relations with the community. One university staff member, for example, completely overlooked the major complaints of community physicians against the university. Attributing poor attendance at some of the university-supported tumor conferences and low referral rates to strictly economic motives, he stated that community practitioners "won't take time out of their office hours . . . . They don't want to lose business."

The medical center clearly projected an air of superiority that community practitioners disliked. While many community physicians looked upon their relation with the university as an opportunity to share its dignity, physicians at the university often seemed to feel compromised by their relations with community practitioners and hospitals, unwilling to concern themselves with the mundane affairs of local institutions. Reflecting its desire to keep aloof of community practice, the university medical center carefully selected the term "relation" to describe its linkage with community hospitals. This concept conveyed the impression of a loose, perhaps even temporary, bond. Cooperating institutions, however, described their ties to the university as "affiliations," at once a more formal designation and a claim to greater status.

The extraordinary status claims of the medical center based on full-time commitment to research and teaching appear historically to have hurt its relations with community practitioners. Informal substantiation of this impression comes from the comments of one long-time resident of the east side, whose father practiced medicine in the vicinity of the Central City University during the 1930s. At that time, the university medical center still employed some physicians on a half-time basis in addition to its regular faculty. The informant recalls frequent, angry comments from his father, who occupied such a half-time position, about his relations with full-time physicians at the medical center. He complained vocally about the unwillingness of full-time staff to communicate and accept him as an equal. The informant reported that his father eventually left the medical center to devote full-time to his practice, never referring cases to the university although making frequent referral to the west side academic medical centers. His explanation for this avoidance of Central City University was sadly reminiscent of community physicians on the east side of Central City during the 1970s: poor communication, nonreturn of patients, unreasonably harsh criticism, and a general feeling of being viewed as a "second-class citizen" of the regional medical community.

In general, community physicians expressed few objections about the technical ability of university staff members or treatment available at the university medical center. Although Table 4–4 indicates that a greater percentage of the physicians surveyed felt satisfied with other referral hospitals more than with the university medical center, the difference is slight. Much greater differences appear in the areas of communication with referring physicians and returning patients to referring physicians for continuing care.

The observation that technical quality of medical care at the medical center receives only minor criticism from community physicians suggests the strong possibility that the university receives fewer referrals than it should. The combination of the convenient location of the university for east side residents and excellent clinical reputation should attract patients on referral from physicians currently repelled by the poorly organized liaison efforts and tradition of academic aloofness of the university. While the university hardly deserves criticism for failing to attract referrals from *every* physician sampled in the Professional Community Survey—more doctors at the hospitals surveyed referred cancer patients to the university than any other referral site—several conscious policies and long-standing attitudes prevent its faculty from achieving this highly important goal of cancer control. Poor communication and lack of sufficient attention to the professional and personal needs of community physicians inhibit many from making referrals that are indicated on strictly medical grounds.

The unwillingness of community physicians to refer patients to the university medical center is tantamount to the underutilization of an important resource in cancer control. If reliable linkages between practice and academic medical centers are a significant element of the social technology necessary for control of cancer and other modern diseases, adoption of this technology has been far from universal in the cancer control program service region. Resistance to forming stronger linkages may be traced to both the university medical center and to physicians in community practice. The medical center evinces no clear willingness to cultivate the ties that would generate additional referrals from community practitioners. Sociologists distinguish between "weak" and "strong" social ties, the former requiring relatively small commitments of time and resources to maintain, the latter requiring great commitments of this nature.[13] Generated through publications and presentations at conferences, extensive networks of loose ties help meet the need of the university for large numbers of research cases by facilitating referral of patients from widely scattered, distant sites. But to serve as a provider of regional services, more time-consuming and intimate strong ties are needed. The university medical center staff members appear to be more comfortable performing the activities necessary for the establishment of loose ties with colleagues. These relationships are more compatible with basic research activities. But other goals of the medical center, whether these are obtaining an adequate supply of teaching cases or becoming a regional center for cancer control, depend on establishing new types of social relations with the surrounding medical community.

At the time this research was conducted, neither the university nor the community practitioner seemed willing to make the necessary tradeoffs required for optimal patient referral. In order to join in an effective regional health care system, physicians at the center and those at the periphery must relinquish important things to each other. The center must renounce part of its traditional commitment to formal instruction and basic biomedical research. Community practitioners must relinquish some of their highly prized autonomy.

Both segments of the medical community must give up some degree of control over their customary spheres of operation to approach modern health problems most effectively.

Despite its discouraging findings, the outcome of this investigation of referral relations within the cancer control program service region is not entirely negative. No evidence of a general conflict between medical "town and gown" surfaced in the research. While community physicians complained about specific features of one major university referral center, they did not question the importance of university-based tertiary care in general. It seems possible that more extensive research on the medical community in the program service region would identify several different networks of physicians, each connecting different segments of community practice with different university referral centers.

Finally, evidence developed that there were great areas of technical compatibility between the needs of researchers and those of patients with at least some of the problems related to cancer. A cancer specialist at the university medical center, for example, repeated his conviction that "good research is good clinical medicine" several times during the course of an interview. By this statement he indicated that research activity may benefit the patient directly, since a well-formulated research protocol exposes the patient to one of two procedures, each of which is considered equally valuable in the medical profession in the absence of further research and both of which represent "state of the art" cancer therapy. Another physician, based in a community hopsital, noted that the social relations among physicians at the medical center, although research oriented, met the needs of some of his patients eminently well. He explained:

> I will refer a breast cancer case to the university under certain circumstances. For example, referral is indicated if there is a multiple systems involvement. Breast cancer may spread to the sternum, or there may be an involvement of the thyroid or other endocrine glands. This multiple systems involvement requires the care of several physicians working in collaboration, since multimodal therapy may be required. *The ability of university-based physicians to handle this type of case is outstanding; they have more frequent interaction with each other and communication among them is easier when necessary* (emphasis added).

## PROFESSIONAL SPECIALTIES AND PERSONAL LINKAGES

While the patient referral may represent the most formal type of interpersonal relationship among physicians, less formal interactions are equally important in the control of cancer and other modern diseases. Less formal contacts may include the exchange of information, either on the physician's own initiative or in response to the request of a colleague, and consultations about hospitalized patients. The physician who requests a colleague to see a patient in a hospital setting may accomplish the same purpose as office-based practitioners who refer patients to each other, that is, "borrowing" one another's expertise. The convenience of merely asking a colleague to see one's patient in a hospital overrides the risks physicians take in making a referral in terms of income and, to some extent, prestige. The communication process among physicians also accomplishes an educational purpose. This form of information exchange may be as valuable as formally accredited continuing education programs or educational outreach offerings such as those of Central City University. As Coleman et al. note, important information related to adoption of new medications depends in part on face-to-face communication among doctors.[14] Researchers on communication patterns in other fields of scientific endeavor have characterized the phenomenon of continuous mutual education as "the invisible university," an informal network of person-to-person information seeking and granting and continuing reevaluation of colleagues' abilities.[15] Processes of this kind are as important to the success of regional strategies to improve health care as the referral process itself. Because these activities are more frequent among physicians and less costly and risky to them than referral, they may amount to more reliable mechanisms to promote appropriate care than either continuing education or referral in the formal sense.

Like referral patterns, many complex and subtle variables appear likely to determine which physicians seek information from others, which receive the most frequent requests, and which are most likely to ask and be asked by colleagues to "look in on" one of their patients. This discussion will address only one dimension of this elaborately complicated set of social connections and divisions, those that occur within and between distinct medical specialties. The "folklore" of medical practice as well as psychological, sociological, and labor market studies suggest that informal communication takes place more frequently within some specialties than others and between certain pairs of specialties more often than between other pairs. These interaction patterns may be attributed to the personality types that various medical specialties attract and to the intellectual traditions and practitioner ideologies associated with each specialty. Thus, surgeons enjoy a reputation for independence and decisiveness, while internists are said to value patience, nonintervention in the disease process when possible, and discursive relations with colleagues. Functional differences may also account for the patterns of informal communication among physicians in different specialties, internal medicine perhaps being a field more open to speculation and interpretation and hence frequent discussion of cases than, say, obstetrics. A full understanding of the informal communication process among physicians would require the construction of a *gestalt* including not only these dimensions, but also factors associated with prestige of specialties and esteem of individuals as cited in the discussion of physician referral behavior.

The present discussion will deal only with the outlines of this picture. It will attempt to demonstrate the major patterns of informal communication among physicians in three major specialties that play important roles in the detection and treatment of cancer. Like the discussion on referrals, this inquiry will ask the major question of whether the prevailing patterns of communication within and between specialties is in fact most conducive to providing appropriate care on a reliable, systemwide basis for cancer patients. The inquiry holds the functional effects of each specialty problematical. While some may argue, for example, that surgeons perform more standardized work and face more explicit problems than internists, they may still benefit from more active communication than seems to characterize their specialty at present. Many practices associated with particular specialties may arise from tradition and historical accident as easily as functional necessity. Where these factors interfere unnecessarily with the learning of new cancer-related techniques and deny physicians access to the expertise of colleagues in other specialties, they hamper achievement of the goal of appropriate care for cancer patients.

### The Professional Community Survey:
### Outlines of Interaction

The Professional Community Survey included a series of questions designed to explore these less formal varieties of interaction among physicians at the university medical center and the hospitals associated with the cancer control program. These questions asked: (1) how frequently physicians asked other physicians in various specialties to see their patients, (2) how frequently physicians were asked by colleagues in other specialties to see their patients, and (3) how often physicians discussed their patients with other physicians in various specialties. Responses to these questions made it possible to determine the specialties whose members tended to interact with each other most frequently and to approach and be approached by individuals in other specialties. Respondents were divided into four major specialty categories: internists, surgeons, radiologists, and others. The analysis then compared the percentages of physicians within each category who reported having "fairly frequent" or "very frequent" contact with colleagues in their own or other specialties.

Tables 4-5 through 4-8 summarize the outcome of this analysis. As in the analysis of referrals, less formal types of physician interaction do not appear to be a random process. Internists, for example, seem willing to approach each other frequently, over 60 percent reporting that they ask other internists to see their patients very or fairly frequently (see Table 4-5). Surgeons report asking internists to see their patients about as often, 60 percent of the surgeons responding to the survey indicating that they initiated contact fairly or very frequently (Table 4-6). Fewer surgeons than internists, though,

**Table 4-5. Contact Among Physicians in Various Specialties: Internists Compared With All Others[a]**

|  | Internists | Noninternists |
|---|---|---|
| Percentages of internists and noninternists asking these specialists to see their patients: |  |  |
| Internists | 61.1(11) | 40.3(27)[b] |
| Surgeons | 78.9(19) | 31.7(19)[b] |
| Radiologists | 72.2(18) | 45.9(28)[c] |
| Others | 44.4 (9) | 20.7(12) |
| Percentage asked by these specialists to see their patients: |  |  |
| Internists | 44.4 (8) | 40.0(26) |
| Surgeons | 47.4 (9) | 29.7(19) |
| Radiologists | 33.3 (6) | 18.6(11) |
| Others | 44.4 (8) | 41.8(23) |
| Percentage who discuss cases with these specialists: |  |  |
| Internists | 77.8(14) | 53.7(36)[d] |
| Surgeons | 78.9(15) | 47.7(31)[d] |
| Radiologists | 52.6(10) | 43.1(28) |
| Others | 64.3 (9) | 47.4(27) |

[a]In this and the following two tables, percentages are abstracted from fourfold tables ($df = 1$) comparing interactions of particular specialists with all other physician respondents. Figures in parentheses represent numbers of individuals in each category who indicate that they engage in the specified interaction very or fairly often. Significance tests are based on $\chi^2$ values.
[b]$p < .01$.
[c]$p < .10$.
[d]$p < .05$.

Table 4-6. Contact Among Physicians in Various Specialties: Surgeons Compared with All Others

|  | Surgeons | Nonsurgeons |
|---|---|---|
| Percentage of surgeons and nonsurgeons asking physicians in these specialties to see their patients: | | |
| Internists | 60.0(12) | 40.0(26) |
| Surgeons | 15.4  (2) | 48.5(32)[a] |
| Radiologists | 73.7(14) | 45.0(27)[a] |
| Others | 30.0  (3) | 31.0(13) |
| Percentage asked by these specialists to see their patients: | | |
| Internists | 61.1(11) | 35.4(23)[a] |
| Surgeons | 29.4  (5) | 34.8(23) |
| Radiologists | 29.4  (5) | 20.0(12) |
| Others | 63.6  (7) | 38.7(24) |
| Percentage who discuss cases with these specialists: | | |
| Internists | 68.4(13) | 56.1(37) |
| Surgeons | 56.3  (9) | 54.4(37) |
| Radiologists | 57.9(11) | 41.5(27) |
| Others | 41.7  (5) | 52.5(31) |

[a] $p < .10$.

appear to make a fairly or very frequent practice of asking others in their specialty to see their patients. Table 4-6 shows that only about 15 percent of the surgeons responding to the survey reported fairly or very frequent interaction of this kind. Radiologists (see Table 4-7) seemed to initiate contact with physicians in other specialties with considerably less frequency than either internists or surgeons; they shared the disinclination to ask physicians in their own specialty with the surgeons, reporting initiating very or fairly frequent contact of this kind with radiologists only about 14 percent of the time.

The reader should view these tables with a degree of skepticism, particuarly with regard to the responses of specialists in internal medicine. Self-reported data of this kind are always open to a measure of distortion by the respondents reflecting values prevailing among significant others. Among the internists who responded to the Professional Community Survey, fewer (44.4 percent) reported being approached fairly or very frequently by other internists than indicated that they approached others in their specialty (61.1 percent) with requests to see their patients. This difference suggests that "sociable" physicians may have been more strongly inclined to partake in the survey and those less likely to initiate contact with colleagues

Table 4-7. Contact Among Physicians in Various Specialties: Radiologists Compared with All Others

|  | *Radiologists* | *Nonradiologists* |
| --- | --- | --- |
| Percentage of radiologists and nonradiologists asking these specialists to see their patients: |  |  |
| Internists | 40.0 (4) | 45.3(34) |
| Surgeons | 40.0 (4) | 43.5(30) |
| Radiologists | 14.3 (1) | 55.6(40)[a] |
| Others | 25.0 (2) | 31.8(14) |
| Percentage asked by these specialists to see their patients: |  |  |
| Internists | 70.0 (7) | 37.0(27)[a] |
| Surgeons | 60.0 (6) | 30.1(22) |
| Radiologists | 33.3 (6) | 21.1(15) |
| Others | 70.0 (7) | 38.1(24) |
| Percentage who discuss cases with these specialists: |  |  |
| Internists | 90.0 (9) | 54.7(41)[a] |
| Surgeons | 90.0 (9) | 50.0(37)[b] |
| Radiologists | 44.4 (4) | 45.3(34) |
| Others | 80.0 (8) | 45.9(28)[a] |

[a] $p < .10$.
[b] $p < .05$.

avoided the interviewers. But this explanation seems unlikely; surgeons and radiologists report receiving fairly or very frequent requests from others in their specialty to see their patients *more often* than initiating such requests. A more tenable explanation seems to be that mutual contact, while a very strong value among internists, is honored more regularly as a norm than in actual practice. The difference between norms and actual behavior that seems likely to occur in this setting recalls a similar observation in the referral area—doctors are more likely to report a great emphasis on referral within their colleague community than to actually refer patients.

Discussion among physicians is the least formal but perhaps the most frequent form that colleague interaction may take. This type of activity involves the least risk and exposes participants to little direct criticism in comparison to referral or asking colleagues to physically see a patient. At the same time, this type of interaction may be the most frequent; it may be observed in any hospital corridor as doctors ask each other questions about specific patients, make wagers on prognoses, and inquire about the benefits and hazards associated with new drugs and procedures. The process is too immediate to be replaced by formal educational efforts, which may work best by injecting more and newer information into the informal exchange.

High percentages of surgeons, internists, and radiologists report fairly or very frequently discussing their cases with other physicians, but as with other forms of interaction, discussion patterns take a definite form. As Table 4-5 indicates, internists report frequent discussions with other internists and with surgeons slightly less than 80 percent of the time. This table suggests the possibility that internists are more likely to discuss cancer cases with surgeons than are any other specialists. Internists are significantly more likely to report such contact with surgeons than are specialists in all other fields. Table 4-6 indicates that surgeons report discussing cases with internists more frequently than with any other specialty, including their own. The majority of surgeons, however, still indicate that they discuss cancer cases with other surgeons fairly or very frequently. Table 4-7 shows that radiologists often interact within discussion networks, but they participate in such activity with other radiologists significantly less often than with specialists in other fields. While 90 percent of the radiologists interviewed reported fairly or very frequent discussions with both internists and surgeons, only 44.4 percent said they very or fairly frequently discussed cases with other radiologists. In one sense, radiologists seem to be among the most active participants in the discussion process, interacting with internists and surgeons in this manner significantly more frequently than do members of other specialties. In another sense, they appear inactive, only a minority discussing cases regularly with members of their own specialty.

Table 4-8 summarizes the patterns of all three varieties of physician interaction less formal than patient referral. The pattern of interaction seems most active among internists. Specifically, internists are more likely to ask other internists to see their patients than are surgeons to make similar requests of other surgeons or radiologists of other radiologists. Similarly, internists are more likely to report fairly or very frequent discussions of cancer patients with other internists than are surgeons with other surgeons or radiologists with other radiologists. Brisk interaction also appears to take place between internists and surgeons, with internists reporting asking surgeons to see their patients significantly more often than do other physicians and internists discussing cancer cases with surgeons significantly more frequently than do other physicians. Surprisingly, very few surgeons report fairly or very frequently asking other surgeons to see their patients, nonsurgeons telling interviewers that they approach surgeons for such purposes about three times as often as surgeons

**Table 4-8. Schematic Models for Three Types of Interaction Among Physicians[a]**

A. *Request to see patients*

|  | Internists | Surgeons | Radiologists | Others |
|---|---|---|---|---|
| Internists | 1 | 1 | 1 | 0 |
| Surgeons | 1 | 0 | 1 | 0 |
| Radiologists | 0 | 0 | 0 | 0 |
| Others | 0 | 0 | 0 | 0 |

B. *Requested to see patients*

|  | Internists | Surgeons | Radiologists | Others |
|---|---|---|---|---|
| Internists | 0 | 0 | 0 | 0 |
| Surgeons | 1 | 0 | 0 | 1 |
| Radiologists | 1 | 1 | 0 | 1 |
| Others | 0 | 0 | 0 | 0 |

C. *Discuss patients*

|  | Internists | Surgeons | Radiologists | Others |
|---|---|---|---|---|
| Internists | 1 | 1 | 1 | 1 |
| Surgeons | 1 | 1 | 1 | 0 |
| Radiologists | 1 | 1 | 0 | 1 |
| Others | 0 | 0 | 0 | 1 |

[a]Entries in cells represent observed tendencies of physicians in left-hand column categories to interact with those in row categories. Interaction pattern is designated as 1 if over 50 percent of physicians in column categories frequently engage in specified types of contact with physicians in row categories and 0 if fewer than 50 percent in column categories frequently interact with those in row categories.

report approaching each other. While the majority of surgeons responding to the survey indicated that they discussed cancer cases with other surgeons fairly or very frequently, the percentage reporting such behavior was considerably smaller than that of internists. Internists told interviewers that they discussed cases with other internists very or fairly frequently 77.8 percent of the time; surgeons reported interaction of this nature with other surgeons only 56.3 percent of the time. Much informal communication, thus, appears to take place among internists and between internists and surgeons. But surgeons seem to be relatively less inclined to communicate with fellow members of their specialty than internists.

Several features of modern medical practice seem capable of explaining the differing communication behavior of surgeons and internists. First, the work of the internist may be more complicated. While the task of the surgeon may be no less—and quite possibly more—difficult and demanding, it seems likely to be more straightforward. The surgeon, because of the highly concrete and immediate nature of the work, seems less likely to need consultations with other surgeons. Surgery is a fundamentally short-term task, and the patient is often returned to the care of an internist soon after an operation. Surgeons, moreover, appear to be highly individualistic, often running their own "shops" within the hospital, and although usually willing to discuss cases with other surgeons, they are highly committed to taking individual responsibility for the required medical work.

To a large extent, the interaction process depicted in Tables 4-5 through 4-8 appears to reflect the usual pathway the cancer patient follows through the medical care system. The patient will first approach the primary care physician, typically an internist. In many cases, the internist will refer the patient to a surgeon for consultation and ultimately for surgery. This step offers ample opportunity for communication back and forth among internists and surgeons. Following surgery, the patient will typically be referred back to the primary care physician or to a specialist in management of cancer cases through chemotherapy, typically a subspecialist within internal medicine. Once again, communication may occur in the form of follow-up reports and discussions, as well as specific requests by internists of surgeons to see their patients or by surgeons of internists for similar services. While the typical pathway by which cancer patients move through the health care system offers much opportunity for communication and other informal interaction among internists and also between internists and surgeons, little opportunity of this nature arises for interaction among surgeons. Apparently, even if the cancer patient required the services of a second surgeon, the surgeon would be approached through the internist to whom the patient had been returned following initial surgical treatment.

The pattern of interaction observable among internists and surgeons, then, appears to have a functional feature. Although traditions and personal characteristics of surgeons play some part in their relative disinclination to engage in the forms of interaction described here, a more important cause seems to be the pattern by which patients move from physician to physician. Even though surgeons seldom ask other surgeons to see their patients, this observation may not suggest any needed modification in the physician community. As long as the internist is the health care system's gatekeeper, he or she will occupy the central position in the physician communication network. On the basis of these propositions, some observers may conclude that surgeons do not need any more contact with other surgeons, and the cancer patient could not benefit materially from increased contact of this kind. The comments of one surgeon interviewed in the study support this position. Explaining why surgeons are less inclined than internists to discuss cases with members of their own specialty or to ask fellow surgeons to see their patients, he noted:

> When a surgeon receives a case, it has generally been already well triaged. For this reason, surgeons have relatively little need to compare notes with other surgeons. A surgical case is generally straightforward, while the work of the internist is typically more complex.

Those interested in strengthening the health care system's capacity to control cancer, however, must take a skeptical approach, looking for ways in which seemingly "functional" detachment of physicians from colleagues in the same specialty may be detrimental to the interests of the cancer patient. One problem, of course, may be in the diffusion of new knowledge. In a field that has received such a large public investment of research funds, diffusion of new knowledge is particularly important. Observers may well ask whether the traditional and functional communication patterns in medicine obstruct this process. Second, investigators must ask whether the lacunae observable in physician interaction may make it impossible for some patients to reach physicians whose unusual subspecialties and skills may be required for appropriate treatment of their conditions. Finally, the disinclination of some physicians to engage in selected varieties of interaction may undermine a critical component in appropriate treatment of modern disease: the cooperation of several different doctors and pooling of specialized medical knowledge in treating cases.

Even more than surgery, the field of radiology appears likely to fall prey to such difficulties. Table 4-7 suggests that radiologists engage in little contact with colleagues in their specialty. While radiologists report fairly or very frequent discussions of cases with surgeons and internists 90 percent of the time—a percentage higher than any other inter- or intraspecialty interaction detected in this study—they discuss cases only half as often with members of their own specialty. Radiologists seem to take a passive role in the consultation process, only a minority of them reporting that they ask colleagues in their own or other specialties to see their patients. The majority of radiologists, though, report being asked frequently by internists and surgeons to see the patients of *these* physicians. Last, and perhaps most important, Table 4-8 indicates that radiologists are the only specialty category represented whose members report frequent discussion of cases with members of their own specialty less than 50 percent of the time. The peculiarities of radiology appear to offer insights into the reasons for physicians to feel disinclined to communicate with others in their specialty or to initiate the consultation process. An in-depth viewing of radiology appears potentially valuable in helping determine whether the interaction characteristics of the specialty are entirely functional or result in obstructions within the process of providing appropriate care for the cancer patient.

### Interaction Among Radiologists: A Functional System or Dysfunctional Survival?

The tendency of radiologists to play a passive role in the consultation process and to discuss cancer cases largely with members of the medical profession outside their own specialty appears to result both from their functional and historical place in the health care system. In a functional sense, there are several compelling explanations of the radiologist's passive role relative to other physicians. For many years, radiologists operated largely as diagnosticians, several steps removed from patient care. Well into the 1950s, radiologists overwhelmingly performed the standardized task of inspecting X-rays and writing reports for attending physicians. With the development of radiotherapy during the 1950s, 1960s, and 1970s, radiologists adopted the expanded function of irradiating neoplasms and instituted the subspecialties of radiotherapy and nuclear medicine. Although the radiologists' role expanded, specifically in cancer treatment, their role as passive figures in the medical network remained intact. Radiologists are seldom if ever primary care physicians. Typically hospital based, they receive patients on referral from internists or surgeons, perform specialized services for them, and return the patient in short order. A surgeon or internist may order radiotherapy, thus initiating an approach to the radiology department. Radiologists, without patients in any strict sense, are not in the position to refer patients to others. They are at the end of the referral chain and perform functions ordered by others in this position.

A long-standing conception of the radiologist's role and personality among other physicians accompanies the type of function they tend to play. According to one study of medical education, the popular student and faculty stereotype of radiology includes an emphasis on money, short hours, and light residency requirements and a deemphasis on direct relations with patients and intellectual breadth.[16] This stereotype received some support from an important study of medical students that found that a high percentage of physicians (about 70 percent) who choose to enter radiology do so rather late in their careers, about 37 percent during internship and another 37 percent after internship.[17] Many physicians interpret these figures to mean that young physicians opt for entrance into radiology after having failed to achieve entry into other, "more demanding" specialties. As a personality type, many physicians consider radiologists individuals who are unable psychologically to deal with the responsibilities and emergencies of other fields of medicine, preferring to occupy isolated corners of the hospital and performing standardized, routine work.

Many recent developments in medicine and medical education contradict this stereotype, however. Radiology has boomed in recent years, becoming a glamour field in modern medicine. With the development of advanced instrumentation utilized largely by radiologists, such as megavoltage equipment for cancer radiotherapy and, of course, the CT scanner, radiologists enjoy new prestige in the medical community. Medicare and Medicaid regulations have also contributed to the increased standing of radiologists among other physicians, allowing radiologists to bill patients directly and resulting in extremely high incomes for some.[18] Perhaps the best indication of the growing importance and prestige of radiology in American medicine is the number of new residents the field has begun to attract. In 1978, for example, more graduates of American medical schools entered radiology than any other specialty with the exception of internal medicine and general surgery.[19] In addition, the establishment of subspecialty boards in radiotherapy and nuclear medicine underscores the expanded role of the radiologist, who clearly can no longer be accused of doing little other than taking and reading X-rays.

If radiology has indeed improved its prestige position and expanded its activities over the past two decades or so, why do the radiologists interviewed in the cancer control program service region still display patterns of noninitiation in their relations with specialists in other fields and disinclination to discuss cases with fellow radiologists? One possible explanation would be that those responding to the Professional Community Survey were all older physicians, who practiced diagnostic rather than therapeutic radiology and were removed from patient care and contact with other doctors. But this explanation is unlikely since interviewers selected radiologists at least part of whose work was specifically cancer oriented. The hospitals participating in the survey were often local cancer treatment centers possessing some advanced diagnostic and therapeutic equipment, supporting radiologists who performed therapeutic as well as diagnostic tasks. It appears that important structural and organizational conditions surround the practice of radiology that continue to perpetuate old behavioral patterns among radiologists even though the breadth of their practice has expanded greatly in recent years.

The tendency of some hospitals to employ few or no full-time radiologists contributes to several of the problems suggested in Tables 4-7 and 4-8. If one or two radiologists are the only practitioners in their specialty at a given hospital, the probability of their meeting either intentionally or by chance may be slim. Isolation from the consulting process may result from the physical absence of colleagues in the same specialty or subspecialty. This problem would be most severe in small hospitals, some of which employ not even one full-time radiologist.

But an equally likely explanation among the hospitals whose staff members participated in the Professional Community Survey—most of these had radiology departments employing several radiologists—concerns the activities that are most directly connected with income and other rewards. All organizations have *reward systems* of some kind that encourage some types of behavior as opposed to others by allocating the highest rewards to those who perform best according to specific criteria. Organizational reward systems may not always be functional. The activities that receive the highest rewards may be those most valuable to the organization at an earlier stage of its development. Although activities that receive lower rewards may now be more valuable to the organization's current goals, the old reward system somehow survives. For radiologists, particularly those specialized or specially concerned with cancer treatment, the reward system under which they practice indeed seems better fitted to past eras in the treatment of the disease than to the needs of patients with cancer and other modern diseases.

The reward system governing most radiological practice has several features that show strong signs of encouraging and perpetuating the pattern of consultative behavior observed in Tables 4-7 and 4-8. A diagnostic radiologist receives rewards in proportion to the number of reports he or she produces on diagnostic procedures, whether X-rays, CT scans, or other techniques. No direct rewards accrue from either seeing patients or consulting with other physicians. For strictly financial rewards, radiologists may benefit indirectly from contact with internists and surgeons. Physicians in these specialties refer patients to the radiologist, and the radiologist must maintain good relations with them to insure a steady flow of requests for his or her services. The reward system appears to be essentially similar for radiotherapists, since they perform procedures at the request of other physicians and typically bill patients directly for each procedure performed.

Every reward system encourages individuals subject to it to develop a "maximizing strategy" that orients their activities toward those that produce the highest and most consistent rewards. Given the reward system governing radiologists, the maximizing strategy is to perform the most diagnostic and therapeutic procedures possible. The radiologist who adopted an ideal maximizing strategy tailored to this reward system would behave quite similarly to the radiologists whose responses furnished the statistics in Table 4-7. This radiologist would, first, seldom initiate contact with other doctors. While he or she would have to converse with them about the cases he or she was sent, this consultation would be most likely to come after a procedure had been performed. Second, the "maximizing" radiologist would have little reason to consult with others in his or her specialty. Because requests for radiological services come largely from internists and surgeons, little in the way of financial return can be realized from cultivating relations with other radiologists. Finally, the maximizer under the prevailing reward system would have little incentive to communicate with or physically examine patients. The rewards come from dictating reports about patients on the basis of highly mechanized procedures and indirectly from maintaining contact with physicians in nonradiological specialties who provide access to patients.

Radiologists interviewed at a professional conference identified several types of practitioners who fit this description. They explained that the radiologist who wished to maximize financial rewards limited his or her time to strictly performing specialized tasks without leaving the hospital's radiology department. Such limitation would produce the highest income per hour, as no time would be "wasted" conferring unnecessarily with other physicians. They specified one type of radiologist, whose behavior mirrored the disinclination to initiate communication with other doctors and discuss cases with fellow radiologists identified in the Professional Community Survey, as the "tram rider." According to their description, the tram rider works at several different hospitals, each of which is too small to employ a full-time radiologist. By spending as little time at each hospital as possible, the tram rider avoids all unnecessary social or professional contact with the staff physicians. Typically a diagnostician, this type of radiologist spends nearly all of the time reading X-rays and dictating reports. Those who adopted this maximizing strategy, the radiologists noted, constituted the stereotype of their specialty as perceived by many other doctors. The tram rider, they explained, could indeed work a six-hour day and earn an income well above that of the average physician.

Despite the negative impression many radiologists hold of the tram rider and other colleagues who adopt similar maximizing strategies, they attributed the maximizers' behavior not to individual greed but to characteristics of the reward system. They remarked, for example, that recent entrants into the field of radiology often desired to change their image among other doctors. They noted that recently certified radiologists disliked their reputation for shyness, avoidance of responsibility, mechanical orientation, and distaste for patient contact. To help dispel this image, they reported that younger radiologists, particularly in academic settings, were beginning to make rounds with internists and surgeons in order to gain clinical exposure and increase their interaction with patients. Toward the same end, they explained that new radiologists frequently sought to encourage other physicians to discuss cases with them through an "open door policy" at the radiology department, letting nonradiologists know that they were welcome to come and discuss cases at will.

But the radiologists who described these new initiatives noted emphatically that those who practiced them often suffered financially. Clinical exposure and enhanced relations with other physicians lowered hourly earnings. As one radiologist explained,

> These initiatives cost us money. A radiologist may spend four hours "bullshitting" with an internist and not be able to bill him or the patient for the consultation. Radiologists who operate this way may end up working twelve hours a day but make less money than a "viewbox reader" who works six-hour days. People used to say that doctors chose radiology because of its short hours in comparison with those of internists and general practitioners. Now, radiology has become more glamorous and better connected with other specialties. But radiologists now often work more hours per week than the general practitioners and internists!

The radiologists who offered these explanations were quick to point out that physicians in other specialties shunned informal contact with colleagues for similar reasons. Noting the negative relation between extended discussions and income (a relationship present in the work of both diagnostic and therapeutic radiologists), they suggested that physicians often avoided attending conferences inside and outside the hospital for similar reasons. As one radiologist remarked, "Internists and oncologists will be reluctant to attend conferences and grand rounds if they lose the income from twenty or thirty patients during the time required." If the reward system—the *financial* reward system, at least—discourages radiologists from conferring with colleagues, it should discourage other physicians as well. Informants in the specialty of radiology suggested that this tendency was exaggerated in radiology because the reward system gave maximum returns to the practitioner who avoided contact with colleagues in the specialty entirely. Similar, though less obvious, disincentives to community participation seemed to govern much activity in other specialties as well.

The pattern of interaction within a specialty is quite similar among surgeons. Surgeons are essentially as unlikely to make or receive requests from colleagues in the same specialty as radiologists are to make or receive such requests from other radiologists. If these loose measures truely indicate the formal referral pattern that prevails within these two specialties, the reward system in each would appear quite similar. The percentage of surgeons who report that they discuss cases frequently with other surgeons (56.3), though, is higher than similar behavior among radiologists, 44.4 percent of whom discuss cases frequently with other radiologists. The difference is small considering the low numbers of radiologists and surgeons interviewed. But the percentages still suggest important differences in the reward systems of radiologists and surgeons as compared with internists. Tables 4-5 through 4-8 suggest that there is a correlation between receiving requests to see patients from others in one's own specialty (an indication of the formal referral pattern) and inclination to discuss cases with colleagues in the same field. The comments of radiologists receive support from the numerical data. That is, the possibility of receiving referrals from fellow members of one's specialty indeed seems to encourage discussion. Looking again at internists, the tendency to receive requests to see patients from specialists in one's own field and to discuss cases with fellow specialists is higher than in either surgery or radiology. Internists seem to have more concrete rewards to gain from such discussion than surgeons or radiologists.

Certain structural features of each of the specialties examined here tempt the observer to attribute differences in interaction rates among practitioners to functional causes. Radiology, for example, may simply be a more standardized field of medicine than surgery or internal medicine. If surgical cases are more straightforward than medical cases, the radiologist's tasks are the most straightforward of all. The reliance of radiologists on fairly determinate approaches to diagnosis and therapy may simply render much of the interaction that takes place among internists unnecessary. The degree of specialization that takes place within the field of radiology suggests that this is true. Until very recently, subspecialties played only a small part in the organization of radiology. In 1968, for example, only 120 radiologists in the United States held board certification in radiotherapy. Radiologists in many locations may still practice radiotherapy without subspecialty certification. In addition, the subspecialties of radiology are few in number. Radiation therapy and nuclear medicine essentially exhaust the list. Based on these structural features, the observer receives the impression that for most radiological procedures, a radiologist will not need to consult a colleague with more specialized experience.

This is clearly not true of internal medicine. Internal medicine encompasses a vast number of subspecialties, several of which have thousands of members. This degree of functional differentiation within the specialty suggests more concrete reasons for discussion and referral than with radiology. The Professional Community Survey, for example, included several oncologists within the category of internal medicine; oncology itself includes "sub-subspecialties" such as pediatric or hematological oncology. At least one important reason for the frequent interaction among internists in this sample was the discussion and referral that went on between internists in primary care roles and internists with subspecialties in oncology. The possibility of referral taking place through active discussion networks, then, is considerably higher than in radiology. Unlike radiology, internal medicine is composed of many individuals with distinct but complementary skills, either formally recognized through subspecialty board certification or informally through the impressions of colleagues.

Surgery seems to fall between internal medicine and radiology in the tendency of physicians to engage in intraspecialty interaction. Once again, this may be attributed to the functional features of the field and associated benefits—both financial and in terms of patient care—that surgeons may draw from interacting with other surgeons. Surgery encompasses fewer subspecialties than internal medicine but more than radiology. If this is an indication of the variation of skills among surgeons, the tendency of surgeons to seldom ask each other to see cases becomes clear, as is the disinclination to discuss cases with colleagues in the same specialty as opposed to internists.

The structural characteristics of the three specialties examined here, therefore, suggest that disincentives to informal interaction similar to those in radiology exist in surgery and internal medicine as well. The same phenomenon seems to occur in all three specialties, with the relatively homogeneous nature of radiological practice exaggerating the disinclination to interact among these specialists. Because the tendency to receive rewards in the financial sense is strongly connected to informal interaction in internal medicine, interaction is encouraged by the reward system in that discipline. The reward systems in surgery and radiology, on the other hand, discourage such behavior.

An adequate explanation of incentives and disincentives to interact with colleagues in one's own specialty, though, requires an examination of rewards other than financial ones among doctors. Earlier, this discussion raised the notion of different cultures surrounding the practice of each field of medicine, with surgeons preferring to take the decisive, active role and internists preferring a less activist approach, letting or inducing the body to heal itself. Interaction patterns are likely to constitute aspects of these medical subcultures, which, in the case of surgery and radiology, discourage interaction among fellow specialty members. A smaller necessity for engaging in such behavior may support a "culture" of self-reliance in both the fields. Again, the comments of a surgeon interviewed during the study illustrate the relationship between the technical features of a specialty and its subculture:

> The surgeon is more independent, more decisive than the internist. His tasks are more pressing. The surgeon is in the operating room with only his residents, maybe spending four hours removing a cancerous colon. He may operate from 8:00 in the morning 'till 4:30 in the afternoon. But the internists have all day to do nothing but discuss cases.

Thus, mutually reinforcing features of medical practice seem to explain interaction patterns that prevail in various specialties. In many instances, particularly in the work of surgeons and radiologists, these factors seem capable of inhibiting the flow of information upon which a successful cancer control program depends.

## IMPLICATIONS FOR CANCER CONTROL

Physicians in the cancer control program service region interact according to a complex and multifaceted pattern. This pattern encompasses several different types of action, ranging from referral behavior, involving formal transfer of patient responsibility and financial benefits, to informal information seeking and giving through brief encounters. The structure of the local medical community channels referral behavior and communication in very specific directions, according to cross-cutting networks within and between specialties, within the community, and between community practice and university settings. Both concrete and nonconcrete rewards and sanctions govern interrelations of physicians. Each group within the

medical community may be viewed as a "social world" in the phraseology of Anselm Strauss.[20] In each such social world within the
medical community, a particular set of rewards, punishments, traditions, and expectations governs the exchange of patients, information, and influence.

What are the implications of these complex medical realities for
the goals of cancer control? Recall that some of the most important
of these goals depend heavily on strong regional integration of the
medical community. The objective of providing every patient with
appropriate care depends on the ability of physicians within the community to maintain knowledge of recent developments related to
cancer and to refer patients to other physicians when necessary. The
observations in this chapter include features of the local medical
community that both promote and inhibit achievement of this goal.

Some of the medical community's central values help promote the
goal of appropriate care. Most physicians recognize the utility of
continuing professional education, an activity that the cancer control
program hopes will bring about widespread diffusion of new knowledge about cancer. The physicians interviewed in the Professional
Community Survey also seemed to indicate that strong values prevailed on referring patients when necessary. Almost 80 percent of the
community physicians, for example, reported that the hospitals at
which they practiced placed strong emphasis on this activity. Also in
the positive sense, no general conflict seemed to occur between
academic and community medicine in the cancer control program
service region. Although the history and organizational commitments of one university medical center weaken its effectiveness as a
regional referral site, area physicians generally expressed no negative
feelings about the benefits of occasionally referring patients to *some*
academic facility. Physicians within the community seemed as willing
to make referrals to doctors at one or another university within the
area as physicians within the university medical center were to refer
patients to each other. These values appear capable of providing the
basis for a successful regional cancer control effort in which patients
reliably receive appropriate care from physicians who keep abreast of
new developments through continuing education or through referral
to individuals recognized as leading specialists.

On the negative side, many barriers block effective movement of
information and patients. Although referral may be a value within
the medical community, it may not be a norm in many quarters.
Physicians may recognize its importance in the abstract and yet
honor it only seldom. The percentages of physicians both inside and
outside the university medical center who usually refer cancer cases

to other physicians are lower than those reporting that this activity is given major emphasis at their hospitals. The interplay of risks, rewards, and values prevailing within specialties keeps the value from uniformly guiding practice.

The observer may legitimately ask at this point whether some of the features of medical practice discussed in this chapter may provide benefits to the public even though they make the specific goals of regional cancer control more difficult to achieve. Central City University, for example, clearly provides an important service to the nation and the world by defining itself as a center of internationally significant medical research. Too great a commitment to building local ties and aiding community physicians, for example, could drain time and resources from the medical center to the detriment of its activities in basic biomedical research. In the language of the sociologist, the university has a *functional* reason for limiting the cordiality of its relations with community physicians—the protection of its commitment to exploring the scientific foundations of therapies for many diseases, cancer receiving special emphasis.

Similarly, analysts might ask whether particular medical specialists may have functional reasons for limiting contact with members of their own specialties. Radiologists, for example, may in fact serve the public best by concentrating on performance of specialized service. Their work, or at least the work of the majority, may simply not require frequent contact with other radiologists. Similarly, the value of self-reliance and decisiveness among surgeons may save the lives of more patients than would the knowledge they could gain by taking a more collaborative approach to surgical practice. The functional approach to medicine has the advantage as a means of analysis of realizing that few activities could continue over long periods of time without bringing some sort of benefits to those affected by them.

The social technology surrounding medical services in the cancer control program service region, though, has many drawbacks for cancer control. While individuals with many types of health problems throughout the nation may eventually benefit from the university medical center research activities, cancer patients now living in the program service region do not receive care the university could provide because its commitments and practices inhibit the formation of more reliable and extensive linkages with community practitioners. While some patients benefit from the radiologist's high degree of specialization and the surgeon's self-reliance, others may receive less effective treatment because these practitioners learn of recent developments in cancer treatment later than they might if they communicated more regularly with members of their own specialty. In

general, the disinclination of physicians in some specialties to interact regularly with others constitutes a barrier to the efficacy of continuing education efforts by the cancer control program or any
similar enterprise. Widespread, regular communication must take
place among individuals doing similar kinds of work for technical
innovations to diffuse far beyond those who learn of them from the
original source.

Vested interest in existing methods of operation, fear of change,
and respected professional traditions all contribute to the persistence
of the existing social technology. Planners interested in promoting
the control of cancer and other modern diseases must formulate
effective means of reducing the influence of these factors. They must
devise sophisticated methods of reducing the impact of status difference between university medical facilities and community practitioners and altering professional subcultures and incentive systems.
If the features of the cancer control program service region are at all
typical of other metropolitan regions, planners must pay as much
attention to social relations among physicians as to establishing new
treatment facilities or regulating the deployment of new equipment.

The physician community, however, is only one of several problem areas concerning professional personnel in the effort to control
cancer. Health professionals other than doctors are playing an increasingly important role in the management of cancer. The relations between physicians and other health professionals may be as
important as those among physicians themselves. Chapter 5 explores
the relations between physicians and the most important nonphysician health professional: the nurse.

## NOTES

1. James S. Coleman, Elihu Katz, and Herbert Menzel, *Medical Innovation*
(Indianapolis: Bobbs-Merrill, 1966), p. 9.
2. Alfred D. Chandler, *Strategy and Structure* (New York: Doubleday,
1963). See especially Chapter 1.
3. Ibid., p. 345.
4. See, for example, C.J. Henke et al., "The University Rheumatic Disease
Clinic," *Arthritis and Rheumatism* 20 (March 1977): 271–278. See especially
cost comparison on p. 756.
5. J.Q. Matthias, "The Control of Cancer in the Future," in R.J.C. Harris,
ed., *What We Know about Cancer* (New York: St. Martin's Press, 1970).
6. J. Wakefield, "The Social Context of Cancer," in R.J.C. Harris, ed., op.
cit.
7. S.M. Shortell and O.W. Anderson, "The Physician Referral Process: A

Theoretical Perspective," *Health Services Research* (Spring 1971): 39-48. See pp. 39-40.

8. Coleman, Katz, and Menzel, op. cit., p. 145.

9. E. Freidson, *Profession of Medicine* (New York: Dodd, Mead, and Co., 1970), p. 151.

10. Ibid.

11. S.M. Shortell and O.W. Anderson, op. cit., p. 46.

12. W.H. Welch, "Medicine and the University," *Science* 27 (1908): 8-20.

13. S.A. Boorman, "A Combinatorial Optimization Model for Transmission of Job Information through Contact Networks," *Bell Journal of Economics* 6 (Spring 1975): 216-248.

14. Coleman et al., op. cit.

15. Diana Crane, *Invisible Colleges: Diffusion of Knowledge in Scientific Communities* (Chicago: University of Chicago Press, 1972).

16. H.S. Becker, et al., *Boys in White: Student Culture in a Medical School* (Chicago: University of Chicago Press, 1961). See Chapter 20.

17. J.H. Knowles, "Radiology—A Case Study in Technology and Manpower," *New England Journal of Medicine* 280 (1969): 1271-1278. See p. 1274.

18. R. Elliott, "Medicare and Hospital-Based Specialists: Pathologists' and Radiologists' Arrangements with Hospitals, 1965-1968," *Inquiry* 6 (1969): 49-59. See p. 49.

19. R.H. Morgan, "The Growth of Radiology As a Major Discipline in American Medicine," *Proceedings of the Institute of Medicine of Chicago* 28 (1974): 255-256. See p. 256.

20. For an example of this perspective, see A.L. Strauss and R. Bucher, "Professions in Process," *American Journal of Sociology* 66 (January 1961): 325-334.

※  *Chapter 5*


# Doctors and Nurses


The cancer control program devoted much attention to nurses. It placed major emphasis on improving the capacity of these nonphysician health professionals to provide cancer-related services. By improving both the nurse's understanding of cancer and ability to perform tasks related to its management, the cancer control program hoped to increase the availability of appropriate health care services to the region's population. As with physicians, the program pursued its objectives through an educational outreach program. Educational offerings included highly technical curricula such as instruction in the administration of chemotherapeutic agents and less formal material related to the emotional impact of cancer on patients and their families. Once again, the program directly reflects the mandate of the National Cancer Act to make the latest techniques in cancer management more readily available to those in need. As in its attempts to strengthen the ability of the physician community to deal with cancer, though, the prevailing pattern of practice and organization in health care delivery constitutes a barrier to success. The social technology that currently orders and directs the efforts of nurses in the cancer control program service region appears to prevent nurses from applying the full range of techniques of which they are capable and limits the ability of instruction programs directed at nurses to benefit the public.

Like other goals of the program, the educational effort aimed at nurses resembles an approach that policy analysts and health planners have repeatedly considered as a solution to the health problems of contemporary American society—the use of nonphysician medical personnel as an answer to the "doctor shortage." Those who advocate the use of nonphysician manpower to meet the demand for primary care often point to an influential study of nurse practitioners in Canada. The personnel in this study held the R.N. degree, and had attended a special training program at the schools of medicine and nursing at McMaster University. This training program concentrated on "decision-making and clinical judgement" rather than procedural skills.[1] The nurse practitioner learned to evaluate each patient's presenting problems and choose among three alternative courses of action: providing specific treatment, providing reassurance without treatment, or "referring the patient to the associated family physician, to another clinician, or to an appropriate service agency."[2] According to this study, the nurse practitioners provided care of similar quality to that of the physicians. Its conclusions suggest an attractive solution to the problems of residents of District 11 and similar areas where lack of sufficient primary care may prevent many from entering the health care system:

> The results demonstrate that a nurse practitioner can provide first-contact primary clinical care as safely and effectively, with as much satisfaction to patients, as a family physician. The successful ability of the nurse practitioners to function alone in 67 percent of patient visits and without demonstrable detriment to the patients has particularly important implications in planning of health care delivery for regions where family physicians are in short supply.[3]

Expanded roles for nursing personnel may be particularly valuable in cancer and other modern diseases. One commentator has suggested that nurses in expanded roles could provide essential elements of geriatric care often omitted by physicians. This author notes that while modern physician training has focused increasingly on specific diseases, that of the nurse practitioner takes place in an ambulatory care context and emphasizes the development of general skills. General knowledge of this kind is particularly valuable in the management of modern diseases (which most frequently strike the aged), because these conditions often involve several different organ systems and include a psychological as well as a physiological dimension. This analysis suggests that patients will benefit from the greater approachability of the nurse practitioner compared with the physician, concluding that nurses in an expanded role give patients "a greater opportunity to verbalize their problems, a clearer comprehension of services available, and a greater appreciation of staff interest in them as individuals."[4]

In cancer, specifically, many observers believe that nurses could play an expanded role in both detection and treatment. The director of a major cancer screening facility, for example, reports that "primary screening for the early detection of cancer can be performed in a most satisfactory manner by cancer detection nurses." He based his conclusion on a comparison of findings by nurses and physicians who examined 4,000 female patients for four types of cancer. For all sites, the physicians and nurses reached the same conclusions at least 97 percent of the time, and in the cases where physicians and nurses disagreed, "there was not a single lesion suspicious for cancer or other serious disease that the nurse missed."[5]

Nurses in an expanded role can contribute much to the well-being of actual cancer patients. Specially trained nurses, for example, can play a crucial part in chemotherapy. Many chemotherapeutic drugs are essentially tissue poisons, formulated to be particularly damaging to cancer cells. Owing to their generally toxic nature, though, nearly all these agents produce undesirable side effects, such as nausea, vomiting, dizziness, hair loss, and in extreme cases, cardiac arrest. Chemotherapeutic agents can be especially dangerous if improperly administered. Many such drugs, for example, are vesicants, chemical compounds highly irritating to the skin. An improperly placed intravenous needle can allow the drug to infiltrate, causing ulcers of the skin that frequently become infected, adding to the discomfort and management difficulties of an already seriously ill patient.

Nurses specially trained in administering chemotherapeutic agents help avoid this class of difficulties. As a clinical oncologist at the university medical center noted, "they have respect for the drug." This may differ from the intern who would otherwise be responsible for administering chemotherapeutic agents. As the oncologist explained, the intern would not have specific training in administering such agents and would be rotated off the medical ward soon after he or she had learned the technique. He noted that the rotation cycle at his hospital repeated every two months and that it took about one week for each new resident to master the technique. "We simply cannot afford a week of mistakes every two months," he concluded.

Nurses can also play an expanded role in care for patients following cancer therapy. One nursing educator interviewed during our research, for example, emphasized the nurse's potential importance in helping patients adapt to changes in body functioning and body image following surgery for cancer. She cited colostomy as an illustration. The patient requires instruction in irrigating the colostomy and must be informed of the proper diet to make adaptation easier. The family must be introduced to the mechanics of colostomy. The patient often requires support in adapting emotionally to changes in a basic bodily function. In a more traditionally medical sense, the patient may benefit from regular observation by the nurse because of the ever-present possibility that the skin around the stoma will become infected.

Finally, nurses are in an especially appropriate position to provide emotional support to cancer patients. They are physically present on the wards much more than attending physicians. The traditions and expectations of their field place strong values on compassion and empathy. They alone have sufficiently regular contact with the patients to learn their particular emotional difficulties and needs. Throughout diagnosis, treatment, and follow-up, the nurse is in an excellent position to assist the physician in monitoring the progress of the case. Proper cancer treatment can be an extremely complex process, a characteristic shared in the management of other modern diseases. Cancer therapy, for example, can involve several different modalities, such as aggressive surgery, with chemotherapeutic and radiotherapeutic follow-up. A course of chemotherapy may itself be extremely complex, utilizing combinations of drugs to be administered at very specific points in repeating cycles. Errors, patient reactions, and complications are possible at any point in the therapeutic process. A very valuable asset for the physician would be a nurse whose training included sufficient knowledge of the most important chemotherapeutic regimens to detect gross error *before* administering mistakenly ordered drugs or to recognize adverse patient reactions and the development of complications.

Central City University's nurse oncology program seemed to aim at educational upgrading for nurses with precisely these goals. As outlined in Chapter 3, the three principal courses offered through the university covered fundamental principles of cancer therapy, administration of chemotherapy, and management of emotional problems of cancer patients. The nurses were then expected to return to their hospitals with enhanced capacity to assist cancer therapy and promote the availability of appropriate care. A successful outcome of these programs would provide encouraging evidence for the practicability of upgrading nurses as an answer to health manpower shortages, the problems of which are magnified in modern disease treatment.

The success of these or any other educational upgrading program aimed at nurses, however, depends on several related factors. Obviously, a stable and committed nursing labor force is required. Educational upgrading makes little sense if nurses leave the occupation before the costs of their instruction have been recovered in service to employers and patients. Nurses must have sufficient motivation to learn new skills. They must be able to integrate the new skills they learn into the multifaceted set of nursing services that cancer patients require; in learning new skills, they must not "unlearn" old ones. For educational upgrading of nurses to produce major improvements in the care of cancer patients, a social technology must prevail that encourages these capacities among nurses. This chapter first asks whether nurses in the cancer control program service region presently possess the required level of commitment to benefit from educational upgrading. Second, the chapter aims at determining whether the nursing role as presently constituted permits nurses sufficient discretion to effectively perform the *variety* of tasks necessary for managing cancer once new technical skills have been learned. Most important, the chapter seeks to identify elements of the relationship between physicians and nurses that affect the latter's ability to develop the professional commitment necessary to become effective agents of cancer control.

## COMMITMENT AND TURNOVER AMONG NURSES

Turnover is a useful though imperfect measure of commitment to a job or profession. The individual committed to a particular organization or calling will remain on the job in spite of bothersome inconveniences and, in extreme cases, great personal sacrifice. The Professional Community Survey asked a series of questions designed to determine how firmly nurses who cared for cancer patients in the region were attached in this restricted sense to their careers. For analytical purposes, it seemed useful to compare the responses of nurses to these questions with the responses of physicians. Many observers report facts suggesting extremely high levels of professional commitment among physicians, such as willingness to undergo rigorous training programs, long hours, and demanding responsibilities. Labor market behavior and other forms of professional activity among nurses that approximated the physicians' would argue strongly for educational upgrading as envisaged by the cancer control program. Substantial discrepancies between physicians and nurses, though, would alert planners to relatively low levels of professional commitment among nurses and to the necessity of finding and altering the factors that weaken commitment before instituting large-scale educational upgrading programs.

In order to help determine the turnover characteristics of nurses specialized in care of cancer patients as a labor force, the Professional Community Survey asked first how many years of experience each nurse had accumulated since graduating from professional school, and second, how many years had elapsed since they each had received her degree. Table 5-1 presents the results of the first question. This table compares the years of experience accumulated by physicians and nurses sampled in the survey.

Table 5-1 presents a discouraging picture to those who hope to invest nurses with advanced training and utilize their services to ease the health manpower shortage. This table shows a fairly even distribution of physicians according to years of practicing experience. The percentage of physicians reporting one to ten, eleven to twenty, and twenty-one to thirty years of experience is approximately equal, with physicians reporting over thirty years of experience falling off somewhat. The pattern of physician experiences presented in Table 5-1 suggests a relatively even rate of entry of individuals into the medical profession over the last thirty years, with extremely high levels of commitment to the field among its practitioners—few, if any, doctors in the present sample drop out of medicine.

Nurses exhibit a markedly different pattern of accumulated experience. The vast majority of nurses sampled in the Professional Community Survey report ten or fewer years of experience. Over 80 percent of these nurses have worked in the field twenty or fewer years, compared with only a small majority of doctors. The differences in reported length of experience between doctors and nurses in Table 5-1 are significant at the .001 level. The table provides strong evidence to suggest that nurses are considerably less committed to remaining in the health field for their entire working lives than doctors, a huge bulge in the category of short experience contrasting strongly with the even distribution of physicians over all

Table 5-1.  Years of Practicing Experience Among Physicians and Nurses[a]

|  | Occupational Specialty | |
|---|---|---|
|  | *Physicians* | *Nurses* |
| 1–10 years | 28.4 | 58.1 |
| 11–20 years | 25.9 | 23.3 |
| 21–30 years | 29.6 | 15.1 |
| Over 30 years | 16.0 | 3.5 |
| 100%   = | (81) | (86) |
| $\chi^2$    = 19.40, $p < .001$ | | |
| Gamma = -.51 | | |

[a]Table includes only respondents with one or more years of experience.

categories of length of practicing experience. The majority of nurses indeed seem to leave the nursing field at precisely the age when marriage and childbirth are most common among young women.

Concluding on the basis of Table 5-1 that nurses did not merit advanced training because they left the labor force within a few years of receiving professional certification, though, would be premature. The figures in this table are entirely compatible with a major change in the pattern of female participation in the labor market since World War II. While it was once undoubtedly true that women generally left the labor force permanently to become mothers and housewives following marriage, many women today either continue within the labor force with minimal interruptions to accommodate these traditional roles or return to paying jobs after the early years of parenthood. As one prominent observer of the female labor market has observed, "most of the growth of the female labor force in the postwar period is due to the increased employment of mature married women, many of whom enter or reenter the labor force once their children are grown or in school."[6] If nurses are typical of other largely female occupations, then, many of them should return to their former occupation after a relatively short interlude for marriage, motherhood, and the initial stages of child rearing.

Unfortunately, this does not seem to be the case, at least among nurses sampled in the Professional Community Survey. Table 5-2 compares the number of years that nurses and doctors report to have elapsed since their graduation from professional school. If nurses in our sample tended to return to their premarriage professional roles following the early years of parenthood, the negative relationship between years since graduation and percentage of nurses sampled

Table 5-2.  Years Elapsed Since Graduation Among Physicians and Nurses

|  | Occupational Specialty | |
|  | Physicians | Nurses |
| --- | --- | --- |
| 1–10 years | 20.5 | 56.8 |
| 11–20 years | 27.7 | 22.1 |
| 21–30 years | 27.7 | 13.7 |
| Over 30 years | 24.1 | 7.4 |
| 100%   = | (83) | (95) |

$\chi^2$     = 27.73, $p < .001$

Gamma = -0.56

would be weaker than the one observed between years of experience and percentage of nurses sampled. To put it differently, the observation in Table 5-1 would be compatible with the frequent return of nurses to the occupation following the early years of marriage. A high proportion of inexperienced nurses could result from frequent career interruptions just as easily as numerous, permanent departures from the field. Widespread reentry, though, is incompatible with Table 5-2. If nurses typically return to their profession following marriage and childbirth, Table 5-2 would show a relatively even distribution of years since graduation, the nursing labor force still relatively inexperienced, but including many older nurses. The distribution of nurses in Table 5-2, though, is quite similar to that in Table 5-1, suggesting that lack of prolonged experience results from replacement of personnel rather than regular reentry.

The nursing labor force characteristics indicated by the Professional Community Survey, then, do not seem to provide fertile ground for significant educational upgrading or expansion of functions. Pervasive turnover of personnel is hardly consistent with increased educational investments or higher levels of responsibility. Tables 5-1 and 5-2 bode ill for the aims of the program for nurses.

The picture provided by the Professional Community Survey differs significantly from that of the female labor force in general during the late twentieth century. Many women, particularly those with professional degrees, return to the labor force after the early years of marriage and child rearing. But the tendency not to return observed here seems to reflect the dominant pattern in nursing. According to comprehensive studies of the female's role in today's labor market, nurses are significantly more likely to drop out of the labor force after marriage than other female professionals. Comparing nurses with the total population of female college graduates in 1970, Altman concludes that "the nursing profession neither loses as many active participants during their late 20s and early 30s nor attracts as great a proportion back to labor market activity after age 35."[7] He reports a similar pattern of labor force participation among nurses and other female jobholders surveyed in 1960.[8] Thus, although there are many more nurses in today's labor force than there were in the 1940s and 1950s, the general growth of the field does not explain away the preponderance of younger, less experienced nurses among those sampled in the Professional Community Survey.

An economist, Altman suggests that lack of sufficient fiscal incentives accounts for the relatively weak tendency of nurses to reenter the labor market following marriage and the early years of parenthood. But working conditions of nurses in hospitals such as the university medical center appear to play an important part as well. A psychiatrist at the university medical center with an especially intimate knowledge of the emotional problems of health professionals, for example, suggested that the tendency of nurses to drop out of the profession stemmed from its stressful nature. He reported frequent instances of drug abuse and emotional distress among nurses, juxtaposing the difficulties in the hospital to the "natural and healthy" desire of most young women to marry and have children. He noted that much of the stress arose from the close physical contact and intimate care that nurses provided to patients and suggested that the unpleasant tasks that physicians delegated to nurses made the role especially difficult. "There's nothing nice about nursing," he commented.

Some of the major stress-producing factors of the nursing role are, furthermore, concentrated in cancer. Cancer patients may present especially difficult problems, as the care for their condition may be particularly complex and the hope for cure problematical at best. In addition, the young nurse may experience particular problems of an emotional nature. As the informant noted, nurses may encounter particularly difficult stresses in caring for lymphoma patients. These patients, generally in their twenties, are easy targets with which to identify. As a result, the nurse develops a need to distance herself from the patient, which may result in a repulsion from cancer-related work or temptation to leave the field of nursing altogether.

The disagreeable nature of nursing—especially related to cancer—cannot explain the rarity of older women in the nursing labor force sampled here. Individuals remain in stressful positions when they have sufficient motivation to do so. One nurse commented during the research effort that she found herself especially *attracted* to work with cancer patients for two reasons. First, she saw the opportunity to perform very important services, which others were reluctant to perform but which patients clearly needed. Second, she commented that cancer patients often repelled other health professionals, both physicians and nurses, because of the difficulty of care, mutilation of patients from surgery, unattractive physical appearance of patients, bad smells, and the like. She noted, though, that the characteristics that repelled others left her a broad area of autonomy, unusual among nonphysician health care personnel. The comments of this nurse were reminiscent of the comments of oncologists who, while dealing regularly with medically discouraging and physically repulsive cases, attained highly satisfying rewards in the form of prolonging life, relieving pain, and achieving difficult cures.

High dropout rates in the sample of nurses examined here limit the immediate utility of educational programs to upgrade their technical skills. But the tendency of nurses to drop out does not indicate an inherently low level of commitment. Nurses in the cancer control program service region, in fact, give strong indications of possessing many of the qualities necessary to benefit from educational upgrading. An understanding of the exact nature of their orientation toward work and conditions on the job explains the tendency to leave nursing much better than the nature of the female sex role.

## THE SIGNIFICANCE OF PROFESSIONALISM

The notion of professionalism encompasses many of the qualities which an upgraded nursing labor force must possess to improve the ability of the health care system to control cancer. Many of the problems related to educational upgrading can be conceptualized in terms of professionalism. Though useful, the concept of professionalism is so widespread in popular discourse that it requires a specific definition in the present context. A clearer definition of the term raises an important dilemma for the planner. Professionalism among nurses is not only essential to allow them to play a more important role in cancer control, but also, under conditions that seem to prevail in the cancer control program service region, can cause difficulties for the enterprise as well.

As defined by sociologists, professionalism encompasses three major values. First, independence of functioning is a key distinction between professional and other types of work. Highly skilled, specialized work cannot be done if the functionary does not enjoy sufficient discretion over the conduct of his or her activities. Professionals in many fields argue that the nature of their work precludes immediate, direct supervision, for the variations and details of the tasks are simply too great to permit outside direction. Some analysts have suggested that the professional's penchant for insistance on self-regulation is primarily a political subterfuge, enabling bodies of individuals claiming a monopoly on expertise to protect themselves from outside criticism and exercise an economic monopoly with the aid of powerful professional organizations.[9] The American Bar Association in the legal field and the American Medical Association in medicine are typical examples of organizations that for one reason or another fight strongly for the independence of the practitioners whom they represent. Both these groups are, in addition, active in certifying individuals to practice professional activity. Self-regulation, then, may have many motivations and forms. But it is a hallmark of professionalism.

Second, some of the most prominent writers about professionals have suggested that these workers, in contrast to nonprofessionals, place strong values upon service to humankind and the communities in which they live.[10] According to these writers, the "service ethic" among doctors, lawyers, and other occupations generally recognized as professional often motivates individual practitioners to lay aside personal interest in status, money, or leisure to help patients or clients who are in need. Often, the desire to serve humankind draws young people into professional training,[11] and the ethic of service to others may be employed by supervisors to motivate professional personnel to improve the quality of their performance.[12] Although the service ethic may be stronger as an abstract value among most classes of professionals than as an actual norm of practice, it is clearly an important part of the professional socialization and day-to-day thinking of many.

Third, professionals are regularly characterized as individuals who hold a strong value upon acquiring and maintaining practicing knowledge at or close to the state of the art. Professional groups continually hold meetings at which new technologies and methodologies are discussed; most publish regular journals for disseminating the same type of material; some theorists identify the desire to advance and spread new knowledge in a particular field of technology as among the key distinguishing characteristics of professionals.[13] Of course, it is necessary to pass through several years of formal and informal education to acquire sufficient knowledge of the esoteric and often difficult material whose command is a *sine qua non* for a professional in any field.

In one sense, independence, service, and infinitely perfectable knowledge may be considered values that draw individuals into professional fields and govern their activities to some degree. But in a more important sense, these items express important *expectations* of those who perform highly trained labor. Young people making career decisions frequently choose specialties that demand large investments of time and money to enter only because they offer opportunities for independent work, service to others, and continuous learning. These features that Americans in the later twentieth century typically connect with professional careers may be considered as both intrinsic and extrinsic rewards for the individual practitioner's sacrifices. Not only are independence, service, and a continuing quest for knowledge pleasurable in themselves to many professionals, but they are also symbols of social prestige and respectability. For many, these intangible marks of distinction may represent rewards of even greater importance than the high financial rewards also associated in the popular mind with professionalism.

Thwarted expectations related to professionalism have typically caused serious problems in the workplace and society at large. The tendency of professionals whose expectations have not been met to affiliate with social protest movements and disrupt industrial operations has been widely documented. Kornhauser notes that large numbers of doctors, lawyers, and scholars in Germany of the depression era joined the Nazis as a means of expressing their feeling that society had denied them the rewards they deserved.[14] More important to the present context, Crozier documents strategies employed by French engineers to gain power in an industrial plant. This writer notes that these engineers, dissatisfied because they are not permitted entry into positions of managerial authority for which they consider themselves qualified, conceal technical information and obstruct innovation in an attempt to make themselves invulnerable to managerial direction and discipline.[15] Other outcomes of thwarted expectations that may have dysfunctional consequences for work organizations may include disobedience, the formation of defensive cliques of disgruntled employees, serious absenteeism, and turnover.

Much evidence exists to suggest that nurses frequently perceive vast discrepencies between their values as professionals and opportunities and day-to-day experiences on the job. This discrepancy appears to be more important in motivating the nurses sampled in the Professional Community Survey to permanently leave the field of cancer nursing than the "natural" predilection of young women to choose marriage and family life over work outside the home. An understanding of conflicts between professional expectations and work experiences in the cancer control program service region helps explain loss of commitment over time and, hence, turnover in the nursing labor force. Of equal importance, these contradictions appear to reflect limitations on the nurse's ability to provide appropriate care to cancer patients while still in practice.

## EDUCATIONAL ASPIRATIONS
## AND ACTIVITIES

The Professional Community Survey included several items related to one of the most important elements of professionalism: the desire for and practice of obtaining new knowledge. Specifically, the survey inquired (1) how many talks related to cancer the respondent had attended in the past year, (2) what topics these courses had covered,

(3) where the talks had taken place, and (4) what topics respondents felt should be covered in the future. Data of this kind are important in determining whether adequate educational resources are available for medical professionals in the program service region. But the data also provide insights into the levels of commitment, aspiration, and opportunity for fulfillment among the region's health professionals. By providing clues to the professional goals of nurses who responded to the survey, these data give the analyst insights into the types of frustrations that motivate nurses to leave the field.

Table 5-3 indicates that educational activity is a common practice within the segment of health care professionals studied here. The table shows that the vast majority of health professionals surveyed attended at least one seminar, conference, class, or talk during the year preceding the research effort. At least according to this rough measure of professional activity, nurses and doctors seem to engage in approximately the same level of participation. Although physician respondents reported attending at least one educational activity 77.7 percent of the time compared with 66.2 percent of the nurses, the difference is not statistically significant.

Important differences, though, begin to appear in more detailed comparisons of the educational activities of doctors and nurses. Physicians, for example, attend more educational activities than nurses. This is true whether activities inside or outside the hospital are considered. Almost 40 percent of the doctors surveyed reported attending five or more talks inside the hospital; only 3.8 percent of the nurses did so. Over 27 percent of the doctors indicated that they had attended five or more talks outside the hospital, compared with 7.2 percent of the nurses. Perhaps the most striking difference between the types of educational activity in which doctors and nurses engage is suggested by the observation that over 68 percent of the physician respondents reported having attended educational confer-

Table 5-3. Did Subject Attend Talks?

|  |  | Doctor | Nurse |
|---|---|---|---|
| Yes |  | 77.7 | 66.2 |
| No |  | 22.3 | 33.8 |
| 100% | = | (94) | (68) |
| $p$ | = n.s. |  |  |
| $\chi^2$ | = 2.08 |  |  |
| Gamma | = 0.28 |  |  |

ences outside Central City, an activity shared by only 14.8 percent of the nurses.

A second important difference between the educational activities of nurses and physicians occurs in the subject matter of the talks they report having attended. Table 5-4 illustrates one major distinction. Physicians are considerably more likely to have attended talks discussing general medical information about cancer than nurses. The general information category covers both research and treatment oriented material; the heading, in fact, was formulated to summarize a broad range of topics that respondents reported, including radiation therapy, chemotherapy, cell kinetics, specific cancer sites, and treatment modalities. While a majority of the physicians surveyed reported attending talks in these areas, fewer than 20 percent of the nurses did so. The table suggests that nurses attended talks on the psychological adjustment of cancer patients more frequently than doctors, but because almost no nurses or physicians reported attendance at such talks, the data are hardly conclusive. Not shown in the table is a miscellaneous category of topics including early diagnosis and detection of cancer; although nurses attended these talks somewhat more frequently than doctors, the difference is not statistically significant.

A quick look at the educational activities of nurses and physicians, then, indicates that doctors are more actively involved in the continuing education process than nurses and that doctors participate more actively in acquiring new knowledge in basic research and treatment techniques, the central concerns of medical professionals oriented toward cancer-related services. This picture is not surprising.

Table 5-4. Percentage of Physicians and Nurses Attending Talks in Selected Topics Related to Cancer During Year Preceding Survey[a]

|  | Occupational Specialty | | |
|  | Physicians | Nurses | $\chi^2$ |
| --- | --- | --- | --- |
| Topic: |  |  |  |
| General medical information | 57.6 (34) | 19.6 (9) | 14.00[b] |
| Psychological adjustment of patient | 1.7 (1) | 6.7 (3) | 0.60 |

[a]Percentages in table abstracted from two fourfold tables ($df = 1$). Figures in parentheses represent numbers in each occupational category attending talks in given areas.
[b]$p < .01$.

Although nurses may have strong professional claims, few students of educated workers would maintain that their professionalism was as strong as physicians. But instead of relatively lower professional commitment among nurses, the Professional Community Survey results may indicate relatively greater frustration in the educational area. The observed differences between doctors and nurses may reflect unmet desires for more continuing education among nurses.

Table 5-5 appears to support the idea that nurses have sufficient interest in continuing education to absorb more of it than they currently find available. This table compares the percentages of nurses and doctors who suggested topics that, though currently unavailable, would be desirable for future talks. Ninety-one percent of the nurses surveyed suggested topics of this kind, compared with 76.1 percent of the doctors. The difference between the two percentages is significant at the 0.02 level. Although the value of the comparison is largely suggestive because of the general nature of the interview schedule item, Table 5-5 clearly does not support the hypothesis that nurses are already offered continuing education resources in numbers and diversity to match their desires. Suggesting more new topics than the physicians surveyed, they appear to be expressing unmet needs in professional development.

Table 5-6 provides clues to the areas in which nurses feel their needs for continuing education are unmet. Most striking is the observation that nurses mention a desire to attend talks in the area of "general medical information" as frequently as doctors. While it does not seem likely that nurses share the physician's level of commitment to remaining abreast of the central technical developments in cancer research and therapy, the similarity of percentages indicating interest in this category suggests that the educational concerns of physicians and nurses—at least within the present, highly specialized sample—differ more in degree than kind. Nurses maintain a level of interest

**Table 5-5. Did Subject Suggest Future Talks?**

|  |  | *Doctor* | *Nurse* |
|---|---|---|---|
| Yes |  | 76.1 | 91.0 |
| No |  | 23.9 | 9.0 |
| 100% | = | (95) | (89) |
| $p$ | $<.02$ |  |  |
| $\chi^2$ | $= 6.25$ |  |  |
| Gamma | $= -0.52$ |  |  |

Table 5-6. Percentage of Physicians and Nurses Expressing Interest in Selected Topics Related to Cancer[a]

|  | Occupational Specialty | | |
|  | Physicians | Nurses | $\chi^2$ |
|---|---|---|---|
| Topic: | | | |
| General medical information | 48.9 (45) | 44.9 (40) | 0.15 |
| Psychological adjustment of patient | 3.3 (3) | 47.2 (42) | 44.41[b] |

[a]Percentages in table abstracted from two fourfold tables. Figures in parentheses represent number in each occupational category expressing interest in given areas.
[b]$p < .01$.

in cancer-related medical information of a scientific nature surprisingly similar to the physicians. The similarity of interest between doctors and nurses in the area of general medical information is especially striking in view of the fact that this set of topics is much less frequently part of the nurse's sphere of educational activity. While Table 5-6 indicates that nurses maintain an interest in general medical information comparable to that of physicians, Table 5-4 suggests that nurses attend talks in this area only about one-third as often as doctors.

Finally, physicians and nurses report differing desires to learn more about the psychological adjustment of cancer patients. Nurses are considerably more interested in receiving the opportunity to attend talks in this area than physicians. The discrepancy between perceived needs and available resources takes a somewhat different form than the area of general medical information. While physicians seem reasonably satisfied with the availability of talks covering general medical information, they do not seem to be concerned with the infrequent availability of talks on psychological adjustment. By contrast, the nurses seem concerned with the lack of availability of both general medical information talks and activities related to psychological adjustment in relation to their interests.

The educational interests and activities that the nurses in the sample express say much about their professional commitment. Unlike the data on labor market behavior, the interest nurses express in receiving continuing professional education suggests that they are strongly committed to their careers. The tendency of the nurses responding to the Professional Community Survey to express an interest in learning more about the central theory and technology of cancer-related medicine suggests a breadth of interest beyond the usual day-to-day activities of routine nursing. The ability of the nurses to name a wide variety of topics they would like to see covered in future educational activities open to them suggests that many have voluntarily thought of areas in which they desired more training. Both pieces of data suggest interest in the occupation and desire to acquire new skills, factors more consistent with occupational commitment than detachment. This observation is especially striking because of the traditional subordination of nurses to doctors in knowledge and rewards. As in the present sample, physicians receive more continuing education than nurses. The atmosphere in which they receive this knowledge is more prestigious (a trip to a medical conference in a distant city confers more prestige than a class held in a hospital seminar room). And the knowledge the physician is likely to learn is usually less standardized than that of the nurses.

While only a minority of nurses in the present sample seem to remain in the labor force beyond the usual stage of marriage and childbirth, the Professional Community Survey yields little evidence to suggest that this behavior results from lack of professionalism. On the contrary, it suggests that the professional orientations of the nurses sampled here exceed the opportunities available to advance professional interests. Although nurses wish to obtain continuing education in several cancer-related areas, they appear to have less opportunity to do so than the physicians. Perhaps this discrepancy results from greater access of physicians to continuing education, either because more talks are open to them, because they alone have the resources necessary to travel to distant conference sites, or because they alone have sufficient control over their work schedules to make time to continue their education. Perhaps the nurse's professional orientation focuses more upon topics in which expertise is less readily available, such as emotional support for seriously ill patients. In either case, the discrepancy between educational aspirations and opportunities to obtain continuing education may account for the tendency of nurses to leave the field as easily as the pressures of marriage and parenthood.

The possibility that nurses may leave the field in part because they find it difficult to fulfill their desire for further knowledge is one instance in which professionalism may create problems for cancer control. A nursing labor force less concerned with continuing education might have less tendency to turn over when confronted with limited opportunities for · furthering their knowledge. A second "negative" feature of professionalism among nurses concerns the social relations that govern the functioning of the health care team. The interrelations between different categories of health care workers, the relative prestige of each, and the prevailing expectations among them may then explain the apparent distaste of older women for the cancer nursing role. The discussion now turns to an exploration of this hypothesis.

## INDEPENDENCE OF PROFESSIONAL FUNCTIONING

The right of professionals to practice according to their own standards and rules is a jealously guarded prerogative in many fields. Even in fields where practitioners must function under the scrutiny and direction of outsiders, individuals early in their careers may expect more self-direction than they actually receive, and persons at all stages may voice claims for more self-direction. While education in a particular body of technical knowledge helps distinguish professional fields from others, independence of functioning is even a clearer distinction. Again, it is one of the principal expectations acquired during professional socialization, one shared by many nurses in the early years of practice.

A series of questions in the Professional Community Survey on interaction between doctors and nurses provided information on the social climate governing the care nurses provide to cancer patients. The ability of nurses to provide care without the direct supervision of doctors would indicate that the expectation of independence was being met. Perhaps the best indication of independence of this kind is the existence of a self-contained community of professionals in which decisions are made by mutual consultation among peers.

In order to evaluate the types of professional relations that prevailed among doctors and nurses, the Professional Community Survey asked all respondents how often they asked doctors and nurses to see specific cancer patients, how often they were asked by doctors and nurses to see specific cancer patients, and how often they discussed specific cancer patients with doctors and nurses. This line of questioning parallels the items covered in Chapter 4. Instead of comparing interaction patterns among physicians of different specialities, the present discussion compares interaction patterns that occur within the medical profession as a whole with the pattern prevailing among nurses, as well as patterns of interaction between members of the two professions.

Summarizing the results of these questions, Tables 5–7 and 5–8 appear to indicate that doctors and nurses perform many cancer-related

Table 5-7. Percentage of Physicians and Nurses Who Frequently Engage in Various Interactions with Physicians[a]

| | Occupational Category | | |
| | Physicians | Nurses | $\chi^2$ |
|---|---|---|---|
| Percentage asking physicians to see specific cancer patient | 74.0 (54) | 49.4 (41) | 8.85[b] |
| Percentage asked by physicians to see specific cancer patient | 61.6 (45) | 28.9 (24) | 15.60[c] |
| Percentage discussing cancer patients with physicians | 80.8 (59) | 63.9 (53) | 4.71[d] |

[a]Percentages in this table have been abstracted from three fourfold tables ($df = 1$) cross-tabulating frequency of each type of interaction with occupational specialty. Figures in parentheses represent the numbers in each occupational category reporting very or fairly frequent interaction with physicians or nurses.
[b]$p < .01$.
[c]$p < .001$.
[d]$p < .05$.

Table 5-8. Percentage of Physicians and Nurses Who Frequently Engage in Various Interactions with Nurses[a]

| | Occupational Category | | |
| | Physicians | Nurses | $\chi^2$ |
|---|---|---|---|
| Percentage asking nurses to see specific cancer patients | 27.5 (19) | 32.1 (26) | 0.184 |
| Percentage asked by nurses to see specific cancer patients | 11.7 (9) | 25.4 (9) | 3.39[b] |
| Percentage discussing cancer patients with nurses | 36.2 (29) | 72.0 (59) | 19.40[c] |

[a]Percentages in this table have been abstracted from three fourfold tables ($df = 1$) cross-tabulating frequency of each type interaction with occupational specialty. Figures in parentheses represent the numbers in each occupational category reporting very or fairly frequent interaction with physicians or nurses.
[b]$p < .10$.
[c]$p < .001$.

activities in isolation from each other. Table 5-7 argues strongly that physicians ordinarily confine their most important communication to other physicians. Thus, the table indicates that physicians are more likely to report frequently asking physicians to see specific cancer patients than nurses are to report approaching physicians with such requests ($p < .01$). Physicians are significantly more likely to indicate that they are frequently asked by physicians to see specific cancer patients than are nurses to report that they frequently receive requests of this kind ($p < .001$). A majority of the nurses surveyed indicate that they frequently discuss specific cancer cases with doctors. But physicians are significantly more likely to say they discuss specific cancer cases with other physicians than are nurses to report that they frequently discuss such cases with physicians ($p < .05$).

Table 5–8 reinforces the impression conveyed by Table 5–7 of isolation between doctors and nurses in the treatment of cancer. Small minorities of doctors report asking nurses to see specific cancer patients or being asked by nurses to see specific cancer patients. And while a strong majority of nurses report frequently discussing specific cancer patients with other nurses, only a small minority of doctors say they have frequent occasion to engage in this kind of exchange with members of the nursing profession. The difference between the percentage of doctors and nurses reporting frequent discussion of cancer patients with nurses is significant at the .001 level.

Sociologists might interpret these two tables as indicating a strong segregation between the roles of doctors and nurses engaged in cancer treatment. To an important degree, these two occupations do seem to conduct much of their business in isolation from each other. An interpretation of this isolation is necessary for evaluating whether the conditions of practice are congruent with the professional expectations of nurses. Several nurses interviewed during the study provided detailed pictures of their careers as clinical specialists in cancer. These explanations provide an understanding of the numerical data on nurses presented above, both related to continuing education and interaction with doctors. The broader picture helps clarify the meaning of the numerical data by sharpening the analyst's understanding of the social context of interaction among professional specialties and applicability of advanced training.

## THE UPGRADED NURSE: SOCIAL CONTEXT OF PRACTICE

The characteristics of day-to-day routines of nursing and ordinary working relations with doctors suggest important difficulties that might accompany large-scale educational upgrading of nurses. First, the basic nursing procedure does not necessarily require contact with the physician. Nurses typically begin their shifts by picking up patients' charts and reading over the orders physicians have written on them. Before starting work, the nurses beginning their shifts often confer with the nurses who have just completed theirs. At this time, the outgoing staff will inform the oncoming nurses of problem cases to be watched on the ward and alert them to the specifics of treatment that the written orders may have omitted.

Little direct contact may take place between nurses and doctors on the typical nursing shift. Attending physicians spend only a few hours per week on the hospital wards, and the house staff is often spread too thin to directly interact with individual nurses for more than a few moments. The minor place that doctor-nurse communication plays in the daily nursing routine helps explain the relative infrequency of doctors' approaching nurses with requests to see specific cancer patients or nurses' approaching doctors for this purpose in Tables 5-7 and 5-8.

This degree of segregation, however, does not indicate the existence of an independent professional community of nurses. While the majority of doctors surveyed reported that they frequently asked other doctors to see specific cancer patients or received such requests from other doctors, only small minorities of nurses either made or received such requests from other nurses. The numerical data articulate well with the general picture of routine nursing activity. Nurses may indeed discuss cancer cases with each other at the beginning of a shift, but they do not rely on each other when a problem arises in administering care. Table 5-8 seems to suggest that except for the initial conference at the chart rack, nurses work in isolation not only from physicians, but also from each other.

Moreover, nurses appear to serve only a minor function as observers of patients for physicians. Tables 5-7 and 5-8 indicate that only a minority of the nurses sampled report frequently asking doctors to see specific patients, and even fewer are asked by doctors to see specific patients. This feature of nursing practice reinforces the impression of isolation of physician and nursing roles.

Just as they do not imply a mutually interacting community of nurses, the numerical data do not imply independence among nurses from physician directives. While the doctor may not be physically present to supervise the nurse, the orders are nevertheless binding. In addition, many formal and informal norms prevail that serve as constant reminders of the physician's authority over the nurse, breaches of which are likely to result in complaints by angry doctors to nursing supervisors and formal reprimands to the offending nurse. The relation of the physician to the nurse is, to borrow the phraseology of one prominent observer, one of "professional dominance."[16]

Knowledgeable informants in the nursing field have connected these characteristics of day-to-day practice with the tendency of nurses to leave the profession earlier or more frequently than they might if conditions were different. One experienced nurse with advanced training in the care of cancer patients, for example, remarked that doctors resent nurses who take the initiative in even obviously useful ways. She mentioned one instance in which a resident had removed a patient's dressing improperly, excoriating the patient and causing unnecessary discomfort. A nurse working nearby offered to explain to the resident a method of removing dressings that would be less painful for the patient. The physician became irate and reported the nurse to her supervisor. "Many nurses begin their careers as initiators," the informant explained, "but receive so much criticism for taking the initiative that they just quit." The informant suggested that physicians praise recently arrived Phillipino and Japanese nurses, not because of greater technical skills, but because they are obedient. Nurses, she explained, may be reprimanded for infractions as vague as "poor attitude." "Why, nurses are flunked out of school for merely being 'uppity'", she explained.

The systematic denial by physicians of the nurse's right to initiate suggestions and take independent action is at the crux of the problems associated with educational upgrading. Again and again, our nurse informants reiterated the theme that physicians did not want nurses to learn any skills that the medical profession did not thoroughly control. "The doctors," complained one nurse, "do not want us to do anything except the routine, mechanical things they themselves order." A nursing educator thought that existing plans to upgrade nursing skills could pose a threat to professional nursing. She said, "We don't like the idea of the nurse's becoming a 'physician's assistant'", referring to the fact that most postgraduate training in nursing emphasized the "mechanical" features of health care such as administering medication, performing standardized tests, and the like.

Other informants with nursing backgrounds pointed out that physicians tend to discourage the unstandardized, person-to-person interrelations that characterize independent and discretionary professional work. Nurses, for example, reported that physicians frequently discouraged them from instructing patients to perform routine self-care activities. One nurse reported that doctors at her hospital objected to her teaching "their" patients breast self-examination techniques. She recalled the doctors' telling her, "they don't need to know that," and "they can't learn the technique." "Doctors," the nurse commented, "prefer to work with machinery whose deployment they can control." These comments seem to reflect a basic conflict that currently confronts nurses.

Nurses fear that their traditional role, characterized by discretionary activity in patient care, is rapidly changing into a set of strictly technical duties. Aside from the discontent that this development seems to produce, greater emphasis in routine technology seems to prevent nurses from applying skills that cancer patients need. As the nursing educator commented:

> Nursing just has a more comprehensive role to play in health care. Nurses have things to offer that the doctor doesn't. The nurse is more prepared to help the patient cope with his illness. She is more anxious to inform him about his ailment and to teach him how to deal with it.

While most upgrading programs focused on imparting specific technical skills, nurses report a growing eclipse of the contributions they themselves value. Informants appear concerned with the shrinkage of independent functions they once performed—meeting the emotional needs of patients and acting as independent observers of changes in patients' conditions were mentioned most—in favor of technical procedures controlled by physicians.

## PROFESSIONALISM, CONFLICT, AND PROBLEMS FOR CANCER CONTROL

Sociologists and other students of the work role have periodically focused their attention on nurses and reported phenomena similar to those described here. Several earlier analyses have noted discrepancies between expectations and job experiences much like those that the nurses we interviewed implied or expressed. The present study has focused on immediate factors of this nature such as the apparent desire of nurses for educational offerings unlike those available at present and problems related to existing interaction patterns between physicians and nurses. With few exceptions, most earlier studies attribute problems such as those identified here to large-scale and seemingly inevitable developments in advanced industrial society. For the planner, this is a disturbing perspective, deserving serious attention.

Social scientists have identified two major themes to account for conflicts in the nursing field. The first is the oft-cited conflict between the ideals of the professional and the demands of the formal organization. Many scholars have suggested that as the large, formal organization arose during the early years of the twentieth century, it created special problems for the professional. Professionalism, as conceived in the discussion above, stresses values of individual autonomy, personal perfection of technique, solidarity among peers, and service to clients. All these values, observers have written, conflict with the needs of large, "bureaucratic" organizations for standard-ized work procedures and loyalty to supervisory personnel rather than clients or professional peers. Research has revealed connections between these diverse imperatives within such varied professions as engineering[17] and social work.[18] Second, analysts of the workplace have postulated a conflict between the individual practitioner's per-sonal desires to aid (and sometimes to harm) the client and the professional value of disinterested service. Although the professional value system dictates personal concern for the client's well-being, it mandates that the practitioner keep some emotional distance, gua-ranteeing equal service to all and dispassionate evaluation of the course of action to be taken.[19] Observation of nurses provides numerous examples of both types of conflict.

Corwin has made perhaps the most detailed investigation of the conflict that occurs between the values acquired in nursing school and the demands of the work situation. As the "basic dilemma of nursing," he cites the fact that although nurses are taught to value contact with the patient, they receive rewards (in terms of approval from immediate supervisors) for committee work, attendance at meetings, and maintenance of charts and records.[20] On the basis of interviews with 295 nurses and nursing students, he leads the reader to think that the most conscientious nurse should experience the most severe conflict. Corwin concludes that nurses who hold strong values in both performing their professional roles and serving the organization for which they work (a "bureaucratic" orientation) are least likely to feel that their jobs offer the opportunity to perform both roles well.

While Corwin places major emphasis on the conflicts between bureaucratic and professional roles, other investigators consider too great a commitment to direct patient service of an emotive, intimate nature as the major problem. The most recent observers note the continuing importance of the service ethic in nursing, one study of nursing students concluding, "All nursing students . . . believe that a focus on the patient as a person is of prime importance."[21] Schulman writes that the "basic psychological orientation" of the nurse as a "mother surrogate . . . characterized by affection, intimacy, and phys-ical proximity" has recently come into conflict with the functional role of "healer," which requires "skilled technical care." Schulman writes that "the trend towards greater professionalization of the nurse continues and with it the nurse as healer assumes greater and greater importance." Schulman attributes much of the conflict in the nursing role to increasing professionalization, concluding:

Nurses . . . are obstinate in relinquishing their ideal. They complain of each development which takes them further from bedside care of patients. They feel uncomfortable and guilty when they go up in the nursing hierarchy for this same reason.[22]

In a comprehensive discussion of these issues, Katz connects both the conflict between the professional and bureaucratic orientations and the decline in opportunity to render direct personal service to dissatisfaction among nurses. Katz writes that the nurse is willing to occupy a low status in the hospital hierarchy in exchange for the right to perform services of a nontechnical nature in a medical world increasingly dominated by high technology. As such, the nurse fulfills many of the functions omitted by scientific medicine, such as communication with the patient's family and serving as a buffer between the doctor and layman, much as the secretary does in the modern corporation.[23] But Katz goes on to suggest that the increasingly standardized and technical nature of modern medicine has greatly increased the abstract, standardized nature of the nurse's role. According to his analysis, the work organization of the modern hospital has made the opportunity to perform this emotive task much more problematical. He writes:

> The modern nurse increasingly formulates her job in clearly delineated tasks. . . . Such formulation promotes clarity and accountability and, therefore, accurate execution of the doctor's orders, the ingredients of rational deployment of knowledge.

Katz connects this process, however, with discontent and the tendency of nurses to leave the occupation:

> All this bears remarkable similarity to mass harnessing of knowledge in factories. The chief difference is that, since factories deal with inanimate products, even greater use can be made of machines. Much of the collation and translation can be done far more efficiently by computers than by humans. Not only are human collaters less efficient, they are also apt to get frustrated and bored with essentially mechanical activity. The solution for many nurses appears to be to leave nursing or to change jobs to see whether a different hospital may offer a better situation.

Finally, the dissatisfaction that arises from the organization of modern health care clearly relates to needs more intellectual in nature than the "mother surrogate" role:

> . . . modern, college trained nurses, having been nurtured and allowed to develop their intellectual potential, find a pitifully scarce market for their capacities in the very institutions that are in desperate need of their talents.[24]

All these analyses connect discontent among nurses with increasing standardization of their roles. Instances of this may appear in the weakening of social support for providing intimate, direct patient care or for exercising intellectual and critical faculties on the job. The contention that greater professionalism itself increases dissatisfaction in an over-simplification of the picture, at least according to the conception of professionalism used here. Much evidence suggests that nurses actually seek higher degrees and positions as educators specifically in order to escape the standardization of roles that increasingly characterizes modern medical practice.[25] In addition, nurses are more likely to identify their chief function as more "professional" than physicians attribute to them. A fascinating study that recently compared the physician's and nurse's conception of the nursing role, for example, showed that the nurses were far more likely to cite nonstandardized tasks of a discretionary nature as their most important activities than the doctors. Nurses, for example, ranked the task of noticing changes in the patient's condition and reporting them as their most important activity, whereas physicians cited "carrying out doctor's orders." The study also showed:

> The physicians ranked nurses' physiological activities higher than did the nurses. Also, the nurses considered their involvement in the patients' self-care and discharge to be of importance second only to their medical activities, whereas the physicians considered these activities to be the least important.[26]

If performance of nonstandardized work activities is an attribute of professionalization, then, nurses hardly seem to reject the role. Rather, the professional dominance of physicians and need for much standardized hospital labor seems to prevent them from becoming fully professionalized although many would like to assume this status. The findings of investigators who connect discontent with increasingly standardized work roles in nursing parallels the comments of nurses interviewed in the cancer control program service area who decry their being channeled into the role of "physician extender."

The notion that increasing disillusionment among nurses arises from inevitable social forces that compel them to perform more technical activities overlooks the fact that many nurses embrace the opportunity to learn more technical skills. The real conflict arises not from the increasing need to include scientific knowledge in nursing services, but from the fact that nurses are often required to perform these tasks in a standardized manner directed by often inaccessible superiors. The traditional nursing function of emotional support for the patient was by nature unstandardized and followed from the great variability of patients' illnesses and personalities. Nurses still wish to perform this and related roles as the survey data on recommendations for future educational programs indicate. The next chapter will examine difficulties in this area in more specific detail.

For the moment, the problems that the nursing labor force presents to the achievement of improved cancer control are twofold. First, the conditions of nursing employment seem to encourage turnover, even among the most professionally committed personnel. In addition to the frustrations inherent in caring for cancer patients, nurses face challenges to their professional values in the form of increasing standardization of their tasks and dominance by physicians over their activity. Second, the standardization of nursing activities and limitation in their discretion on the job threaten to undermine important patient care activities.

Although serious, the problems that the social relations surrounding nursing present do not appear to be insoluable. Several features of modern medical practice, in fact, provide nurses with opportunities to carve areas of discretion for themselves out of the official authority system. The essentially flexible nature of these relations receives major emphasis in the work of Strauss, who characterizes the interrelations between doctors and nurses as a "negotiated order."[27] Because of the uncertainties inherent in serious illness, courses of action and the right to decide important issues are constantly being negotiated and renegotiated among physicians, nurses, patients, and all other actors involved in the health care process. Much of the problem that stands in the way of educational upgrading for nurses seems reducible to the relative power and privilege of physicians and nurses. Perhaps the best solution to this problem is to provide the nurse with more "bargaining chips" in the negotiation process. Unlike the impressions of some investigators of the nursing role, professionalization may be the very phenomenon that will give the nurse sufficient confidence and social support to develop a more satisfying work role out of the existing pattern of social relations.

Like Chapter 4, this chapter has focused on structural features of health care. Chapter 4 suggests that socially enforced lines of communication and boundaries among physicians are capable of channeling flows of knowledge and patients in directions that are not necessarily the most conducive to improved cancer control. The present chapter has identified patterns of communication and association between physicians and nurses which appear capable of (1) preventing nurses from applying their knowledge most effectively, and (2) driving highly professionalized nurses out of the field. These structural features outline the mechanisms by which key cancer-related health services are delivered in the cancer control program service region. They reflect important elements of the social technology that translates medical knowledge into concrete service. Chapters 4 and 5 have implied that these structural features stand in the way of the goals of the cancer control program by limiting the regional population's access to appropriate service. Chapters 6 and 7 provide more direct evidence that these and similar structural features prevent the public from receiving the full benefits of cancer control.

## NOTES

1. W.D. Spitzer et al., "The Burlington Randomized Trial of the Nurse Practitioner," *New England Journal of Medicine* 290 (January 31, 1974): 252-256. See p. 252.

2. Ibid., p. 252.

3. Ibid., p. 255.

4. R.S. Pomerantz, "The Nurse in an Expanded Role: A Proposed Solution to the Problems of Geriatric Care," *Journal of Chronic Disease* 20 (1975): 561-563. See p. 562.

5. D.G. Miller, "What is Early Detection Doing," *Cancer* 37 (1976): 246-432. See p. 430.

6. I.V. Sawhill, "Perspectives on Women and Work in America," in J.J. O'Toole, ed., *Work and the Quality of Life* (Cambridge, Mass.: MIT Press, 1975), pp. 88-105.

7. Stuart Altman, *Present and Future Supply of Registered Nurses* (Washington, D.C.: U.S.D.H.E.W., Publication No. (NIH) 72-134, 1971), p. 103.

8. Ibid., p. 102.

9. An instance of this in the area of health care is described in J.G. Burrows, *AMA: Voice of American Medicine* (Baltimore: Johns Hopkins Press, 1963). See especially pp. 1-51.

10. The service ethic among professionals receives major emphasis in W.J. Goode, "The Theoretical Limits of Professionalization," in A. Etzioni, ed., *The Semi-Professions and Their Organization* (New York: The Free Press, 1969), pp. 266-313, and in T. Parsons, *The Social System* (New York: The Free Press, 1965), especially Chapter 10.

11. An excellent example of this process occurs among teachers, as described by D.C. Lortie in *Schoolteacher* (Chicago: University of Chicago Press, 1975). Chapter 2 is especially useful in describing values affecting teacher recruitment.

12. Scott describes a method known as "therapeutic supervision" by which supervisors in a social work agency reawaken the values ideally utilized in social work practice among their subordinates. See "Professional Employees in a Bureaucratic Structure" in Etzioni, op. cit.

13. H.L. Wilensky, "The Professionalization of Everyone?" *American Journal*

*of Sociology* 70 (September 1964): 137-158. See especially p. 153 for material on orientation to continuing education through journal readership.

14. W. Kornhauser, *The Politics of Mass Society* (New York: The Free Press, 1959), p. 188.

15. M. Crozier, *The Bureaucratic Phenomenon* (Chicago: University of Chicago Press, 1963), pp. 112-144.

16. E. Freidson, *Professional Dominance: The Social Structure of Medical Care* (New York: Atherton Press, 1970).

17. One of many examples in the engineering field is described by T. La Porte "Conditions of Strain and Accommodation in Industrial Research Organizations," *Administrative Science Quarterly* 10 (1965): 21-38.

18. Scott, op. cit.

19. Parsons, op. cit.

20. R.G. Corwin, "The Professional Employee: A Study of Conflict in Nursing Roles," *American Journal of Sociology* 66 (1961): 604-615.

21. S.J. Jones and Paul K. Jones, "Nursing Student Definitions of the Real Nurse," *Journal of Nursing Education* 16 (April 1977): 15-21.

22. S. Schulman, "Basic Functional Roles in Nursing: Mother Surrogate and Healer," in E. Gartly Jaco, ed., *Patients, Physicians, and Illness* (Glencoe, Ill.: The Free Press, 1958), pp. 528-537. See p. 536 for quotation.

23. For comprehensive discussion of the nontechnical, emotive, buffer roles played by females in the modern corporation, see R.M. Kanter, *Men and Women of the Corporation* (New York: Basic Books, 1977), Chapter 4.

24. F.E. Katz, "Nurses," in A. Etzioni, op. cit., pp. 54-81.

25. A discussion of the correlates of status attainment by Vaughn and Johnson suggests strong correlations between continuing education, advanced degrees, and nonstaff nursing positions. One convincing interpretation of this relationship is that nurses look to education as an avenue of occupational mobility toward alternative positions removed from bedside nursing. See J.C. Vaughn and W.L. Johnson, *The Process of Attainment of Supervisory and Leadership Positions in Nursing: A Multivariate Analysis*, presented at the 72nd Annual Meeting of the American Sociological Association, Chicago, September 5-9, 1977.

26. D.M. Ambrose, "Physicians and Nurses Rank Importance of Nursing Activities," *Hospitals* 51 (November 1977): 115-118. See p. 116 for quotation.

27. A.L. Strauss, L. Schatzman, and R. Bucher, "Negotiated Order and the Coordination of Work," in A.L. Strauss, ed., *Professions, Work, and Careers* (San Francisco: The Sociology Press, 1971).

# Chapter 6

# Emotional Needs of Patients and Professional Practice

One particularly important activity in the care of patients with cancer and other modern diseases is emotional and psychological support. In an age when concrete therapeutic technology receives predominant emphasis, emotional support may appear to many as an overly humanistic concept whose value to the patient is impossible to demonstrate if not entirely insubstantial. But emotional support is critical for cancer patients who must often make difficult adjustments in thought and style of life following major medical procedures or in anticipation of death. Social technology is particularly important in promoting or reducing the health care system's ability to provide cancer patients with the emotional support they need. Elements of the social technology surrounding cancer treatment such as professional socialization, interrelations, values, and scheduling priorities appear to influence the ability of the health care provider to help cancer patients adjust emotionally to their illness. By identifying features of the social technology that limit the patient's access to support of this kind, the present chapter demonstrates the manner in which established methods of providing health care can undermine the goals of cancer control or similar innovations in health care delivery.

Researchers on the emotional needs of cancer patients have identified several major problems that health professionals everywhere face in dealing with the illness. The most obvious problem is the need of the professional to provide cancer patients with sufficient understanding and comfort to adjust to major emotional traumas and the possibility or immediate threat of death. But cancer patients appear to require adequate emotional support for more concrete reasons as well. Effective medical care of a purely physiological nature may depend on a sufficiently high level of emotional support. Cobb, for example, suggests that the physician's sidestepping of emotional issues in patient care may hamper medical treatment by inducing the patient to go "doctor shopping" in search of more empathetic treatment or to seek out quack practitioners.[1] The unwillingness or inability of professionals to provide patients with emotional support doubtlessly contributes to problems such as denial of illness, delay in seeking treatment, and noncompliance with medical directives among cancer victims. By eclipsing the emotional element in illness, modern medicine may cure the patient's physical illness but leave the patient debilitated in other important respects. Many factors in the education of practitioners and the organization of modern medical care deter professionals from assuming the emotional support role comfortably or effectively, an unfortunate reality because the patient both expects and needs this kind of assistance. As Holland writes, "the patient . . . has the right to expect the physician to be competent in offering constructive emotional support . . . no patient wants all art and no science in his medical care, but by the same token, not 'all science and no art'."[2]

The Professional Community Survey attempted to evaluate the ability of health care facilities associated with the Central City University Cancer Control Program to provide cancer patients with adequate emotional support. Because quantitative outcome data are nearly impossible to obtain in this area, the survey aimed at indirect evidence to help judge whether cancer patients could find reliable sources of emotional support within the health care system. Survey questions related to emotional support concentrated on determining (1) whether the health care system—or, rather, the specific fragment of the system examined here—assigned the occupants of particular roles the task of providing emotional support to cancer patients; (2) how well different members of the health care team felt their education prepared them to meet the patient's emotional needs; and (3) how different classes of professionals who cared for cancer patients viewed the problem of emotional support. As in earlier chapters, the comments of health professionals in face-to-face interviews provided guidelines for interpreting the quantitative findings. As in Chapter 7, which is next, the present discussion attempts to illustrate the manner in which patterns of social relations surrounding medical services may affect the ability of health care organizations to deal effectively with the special problems of cancer and other modern diseases. Reflecting the intention of the book as a whole, Chapter 6 strives to present a strong hypothesis about social factors affecting the availability of emotional support for cancer patients. While the data presented in this chapter do not *prove* general principles about health care in the contemporary United States, they should direct the attention of analysts and planners to features of existing social technology likely to undermine the goals of modern disease control in many specific regional and organizational settings.

## THE IMPORTANCE OF EMOTIONAL SUPPORT

The concept of emotional support may, unfortunately, seem insubstantial and superfluous to some analysts of health care. The term's humanistic ring and connotation of "liberal arts" rather than "scientific" skills may tempt critics to label the function a "frill" that, although perhaps acceptable in an economy of abundance, represents waste in periods of retrenchment. This interpretation of emotional support services is extremely dangerous to effective health planning in both cancer and other modern diseases. A few examples of the integral part emotional support plays in effective cancer treatment should invalidate this interpretation in the minds of most observers. Lack of adequate emotional support can have highly concrete and extremely detrimental consequences for the victims of cancer and other modern diseases.

The most striking demonstration of the importance of emotional support in cancer treatment occurs among patients in terminal stages of the disease. Death is an ultimately unavoidable problem of the species, a trauma shared by all humankind. Among dying patients, health care professionals may assume the function that the clergy played in less secular times in dealing with the problem of human mortality. Even when it is encountered in its most treatable forms, however, cancer presents a special set of difficulties for emotional adjustment. Many forms of cancer are difficult to diagnose, and even after physicians have confirmed the presence of the disease, they may find it extremely difficult to determine how far it has spread. This degree of uncertainty has emotional consequences for patients, some of whom may convince themselves they will recover despite indications to the contrary, others fearing the worst despite hopeful signs. In both instances, an atmosphere of extreme anxiety is likely to prevail. In addition, modern therapeutic procedures often delay an inevitable death for years or require patients to adjust to greatly altered body functions as a result of medical intervention. Adaptation to either condition is often extremely difficult.

The level of anxiety that the cancer patient experiences and the degree to which the patient can successfully adapt to the illness (or the consequences of successful therapy) may depend as much on the approach of health professionals as the organic nature of the disease. The skill and understanding with which health professionals govern their relations with patients condition the cancer victim's adaptation to the disease. The two most important features of the doctor-patient relationship in cancer—the giving of diagnoses and information about changed body functioning following treatment—help illustrate the importance of emotional support for the success of the most concrete aspects of cancer therapy.

### The Giving of Information

Informing the patient of the presence of a malignancy is the most fundamental and often the most difficult feature of the doctor-patient relationship. The process of communicating this information is complex, and its mishandling can adversely affect both the quality of the doctor-patient relationship and the quality of life experienced by the patient. The appropriate amount of knowledge to be imparted and the methods by which the task should be performed differ strongly from patient to patient. An emotionally strong individual may be able to tolerate more direct information than a patient with obvious emotional difficulties. Whatever the emotional resources of the patient, however, the physician must often inform the patient of this life-threatening condition in order to secure agreement to submit to therapy and, for terminal illness, to put his or her affairs in order.

The process that some physicians use to inform patients of a threatening diagnosis or prognosis illustrates the sensitivity that the process may require. If the physician feels it wise to inform the patient, he or she is likely to begin with the least fear-arousing statement possible and escalate to more explicit language if subtle suggestion proves ineffective. The physician wishing to spare the patient as much emotional stress as possible may, for example, employ half-truths or euphemisms as long as practicable. One keen observer of British medicine reports the following communications from doctors to indirectly inform the patient of the presence of a malignancy and the need for treatment:

> Well, there is an ulcer there as you can see. Our tests showed that there is a bit of activity about it. So we have decided to remove it in case it becomes dangerous in time.
>
> Well, it's a little growth and we've decided to remove it in case it becomes troublesome.[3]

This study also indicated that physicians may go to great lengths to reassure the patient that a procedure has been effective. Often this takes the form of omitting expressions of doubt and pessimistic impressions from the communication, even when cause for pessimism exists:

Yes (you have breast cancer), but it's treatable and we should be able to cure it. I wouldn't worry about it. There are many women going around without a breast, you know.

Well yes, I suppose you could call it cancer. But this doesn't mean that you should worry about it. It's a curable kind. We have removed it all and we expect you to have no more trouble. So I don't think you have any cause to worry about it.[4]

The study indicated that physicians understated the seriousness of the patient's condition as often as possible. Even under the pressure of possible refusal of treatment, physicians tended to avoid the word "cancer," saving specific reference to malignancy as a last resort. The experience of one doctor with a patient faced with an especially distasteful course of therapy illustrates the gradations of alarm physicians will express to patients under varying conditions:

Give them every chance, apply considerable pressure, use all these vague terms. I'd one patient recently who went through all these stages . . . he had cancer of his penis. And, in the end I said, "Do you know what this is?" And he said "No." I told him, "This is cancer of the penis. It's going to get bigger, it's going to obstruct your water, it's going to get painful and it's going to spread to the glands. And yet, if you just come in and have it operated on, your chances of cure are 99 percent." And he said, "All right, I'll come in." And he had the (operation).[5]

Physicians in the United States are also reported to minimize the emotional impact of cancer diagnosis by understating its seriousness and often not telling the patient he or she has cancer. A 1953 study of physicians in the Philadelphia area revealed that 69 percent of the respondents seldom or never told their patients when they had cancer. The study suggested that physicians who treated more serious malignancies were less likely to tell their patients the true nature of their illness than doctors who treated relatively tractable forms of the disease.[6] A study conducted in 1960 indicated similar findings. A survey of 5,000 physicians in the United States indicated that only 16 percent always informed their patients who had "incurable cancer," while 22 percent *never* revealed such a diagnosis to their patients.[7] The Professional Community Survey, indicating that 20 percent of the physicians surveyed expressed fundamental disagreement with the statement that "cancer patients should be told their diagnosis as soon as possible," suggests that physicians have by no means abandoned this way of dealing with the issue.

Physicians typically explain their reluctance to reveal cancer diagnoses—especially diagnoses of incurable, terminal illness—in terms of the need to avoid adverse emotional reactions from the patient. In an outstanding study of physician attitudes toward informing patients that they have cancer, Oken reports that the argument against revealing diagnoses of malignancies "centers on the anticipation of profoundly disturbing psychological effects."[8] By telling patients they have cancer, many physicians apparently fear the release of emotions that they will be unable to handle. As Davis notes in another study of the physician-patient relationship in cancer, "Presenting so unwelcome a prospect (as a prognosis of death, demise, or permanent disability) is bound to meet with a strong and, according to many of the personnel, unmanageable emotional reaction."[9] The strategy of avoiding transmission of alarming information to seriously ill patients is not new, and it is often cited as a medically necessary expedient. Physicians have felt so strongly that information about threatening possibilities may adversely affect the patient's response to therapy that they have introduced the argument to defend themselves in malpractice suits charging them with failure to obtain adequate informed consent.[10]

Many individuals, quite possibly the majority of human beings, find it difficult or impossible to acknowledge that they are seriously ill or that death may not be far off. Psychologists have characterized this approach to major threats to life and well-being as "denial," a phenomenon that occurs very frequently among cancer patients. Numerous physicians utilize this apparently natural human tendency to facilitate their own wish to avoid informing the patient of a cancer diagnosis. McIntosh, for example, concludes his study by stating that only a minority of the patients he studied "sought to eradicate their uncertainty by trying to find out *the truth* about their condition," while the majority "preferred uncertainty to knowing because it was precisely that uncertainty which afforded them hope." He characterizes the needs of the doctor and patient as quite compatible, with the physician's circumventing the emotional management problem by refraining from providing the patient disturbing information and the patients' seeking "exclusively information which would reinforce an optimistic conception of their condition."[11] McIntosh ends his book with the statement:

This has been a tale of hope: the doctors' overriding concern to leave the patient with hope; the desperate need of most patients to retain some semblance of hope; the clinging to hope despite evidence to the contrary; and the desperate search for signs of hope where, very often, little existed.[12]

But despite the apparently humane nature of the cancer patient's tacit agreement with the physician that diagnoses and prognoses remain unstated, observers have many reasons to suspect that the strategy has damaging effects in some instances. First, uncertainty itself may produce high levels of anxiety among cancer patients. McIntosh himself recognizes this possibility, noting that some patients who are not told the nature of their illness "may feel they are not being told because the prognosis is bad," and, for many patients, "the uncertainty created through not telling . . . may give rise to greater anxiety than would a policy geared to informing them that they have the disease."[13] Other research tends to confirm this hypothesis. A study focusing on the social and psychiatric aspects of cancer, for example, reports that patients who had not been informed of their diagnoses manifested more symptoms of emotional disturbance than those who had been informed.[14] Furthermore, the atmosphere of uncertainty seems capable of producing sufficient anxiety to adversely affect the quality of interaction between patients and their loved ones. One example in a study of terminal cancer patients describes a woman who:

. . . suspected the "worst" about her husband. However, she was sure that her husband was not aware of the seriousness of his condition. She lived in a constant state of anxiety and apprehension that her suspicions might "slip out." In order to ensure against this happening, she studiously avoided talking with any of her husband's doctors or nurses. Even though she would have liked to know what to expect, she used ignorance as a shield behind which her knowledge could be hidden. She avoided discussions with her husband about deaths of friends, illness in friends or family, and any situation which might intimate how ill he was, even if only by association. The avoidance meant that she had to virtually avoid her husband. . .[15]

The woman in this example strove to avoid "disturbing" her husband by transmitting knowledge of his condition to him, but at the price of limiting her contact with him. The observer must ask a serious question about this and similar instances in which the patient's emotional state is "protected." Are the emotional benefits that such strategies bring to cancer victims worth the price they pay in lost companionship and the opportunity to discuss and prepare for death with loved ones?

The ability of patients to informally determine the nature of their illness and their prognosis raises additional questions about the wisdom of tacit agreements among patients, relatives, and doctors to keep medical information secret as a method of handling the emotional stress related to cancer. McIntosh describes several patients who were able to determine that they had cancer by realizing the specialty of physicians to whom they were referred. Others compared their symptoms with those of patients in the same ward who knew they had cancer. Still others compared the treatment they were receiving with those described by patients who knew they had cancer, making surprisingly accurate inferences. An informal information network on hospital wards transmitted news about planned procedures, test results, and diagnoses. Finally, patients often became aware that they had terminal malignancies because they were constantly reentering the hospital but were making no perceivable improvements.[16] The contradiction between official secrecy and the patients' actual knowledge of their conditions becomes particularly striking in the light of numerical evidence that such knowledge is extremely widespread among cancer victims. Peck, for example, reports that 80 percent of the cancer patients he studied were able to name their diagnosis.[17]

The classical disinclination of the physician to inform the patient of a diagnosis of cancer or an unfavorable associated prognosis, then, represents a faulty strategy for managing emotional needs in many cases. Few, or course, would argue that physicians would deal with the emotional problems of cancer patients more appropriately by telling all cancer victims their complete diagnoses and prognoses. But in the many instances when patients genuinely wish to learn their diagnoses, have already figured it out on their own, or suffer extreme anxiety or social debilitation because of uncertainty, there is little basis on which to withhold the information.

Optimal management of the emotional stress related to patients' realization that they have a life-threatening illness requires two specific skills: first, the ability to determine whether and how much patients want to know about their condition, and, second, the ability to help patients integrate the knowledge into their conceptual apparatus and adjust to its implications. Neither of these two skills is standardizable, both depending to an important degree on clinical knowledge and experience. In this sense, they resemble many of the skills physicians already employ in their treatment of physiological problems. To an important extent, physicians believe this experientially based understanding superior to not only abstract considerations posed in textbooks, but even to scientifically verified knowledge.[18] In this vein, one observer has summarized the principles of deciding whether or not to inform a cancer patient of the illness:

> . . . with experience an observant clinician acquires increasing insight into human nature and becomes intuitively aware of what the person under his care would like to know.[19]

If asked by a layman, most physicians would undoubtedly express agreement with this statement.

If transmitting this type of knowledge seems difficult, though, actually helping the patient deal with the knowledge is even more challenging. An important study on awareness among cancer patients makes this plain, concluding that receiving information alone does not help the patient deal with the disease. The study contradicts the working assumption among many physicians that "explicit information in diagnosis from a reputable source results in . . . conscious integration of all pertinent information leading to appropriate behavior patterns including the recognition of imminent death."[20]  In this way, the patient may learn that he or she is terminally ill yet still exhibit all the manifestations of a person who has blocked the information out of consciousness. The patient may still avoid discussion of death (refusing social contact to facilitate denial), refrain from settling his or her affairs, and adopt so hostile and depressed an attitude as to markedly lower the quality of life during his or her remaining years. Far from a simple imparting of information, informing the patient of the illness often requires assistance of the process by which the patient "works through" the knowledge in the Freudian sense, adjusting his or her plans and feelings to discouraging yet often unchangeable realities. This process requires activity by the physician that is both more complex and personally involving than mere transmission of facts. As Peck has observed:

> The recurrent question of to tell or not to tell the patient he has cancer seems almost academic in the light of the finding that 80 percent of these patients already know their diagnosis. Emphasis should be shifted to how the patient is integrating the existing knowledge of his diagnosis. . . . The physician must be in touch with his own reactions to the disease itself, to treatment and to his own role as the physician of the patient with cancer.[21]

### Adjustment to Therapeutic Procedures

Although most social, psychological, and psychiatric studies of cancer patients have focused upon informing the patient of life-threatening illness, learning to live with the disease or medical interventions associated with it is of equal importance. Advances in cancer therapy and increases in the life expectancy of cancer victims have come, in part, at the price of drastically altered life-styles for the recipients of the new treatments. Many surgical interventions become the functional equivalents of chronic illnesses themselves. Patients, for example, may receive mastectomies for breast cancer; they may undergo colostomies for colon and rectal malignancies; they may be forced to submit to amputation for malignant melanomas. All these procedures may alter the patients' image of his physical appearance and social acceptability in drastic ways; they may affect his ability to hold a job; they may destabilize family relationships. While procedures such as these are often necessary to insure the physical survival of patients, they may produce survival at a very unsatisfying level or, taking the patients' satisfaction and quality of life into account, an entirely marginal one. Difficult and costly surgery may be unwise if its consequences include extreme depression, social withdrawal, and, in the most extreme cases, suicide. A striking instance cited by McIntosh illustrates the tradeoffs between physical survival and emotional well-being that cancer therapy may involve. In an interview, a physician described a second case involving cancer of the penis:

> (this was another) young man who . . . had cancer of the penis . . . which, when you think that we see one or two every three years, is rather extraordinary . . . who flatly refused (treatment). He was Dr. McDonald's patient and he told him what it was and what would happen. He again refused. He was a young chap and this was the final indignity—to have his penis cut off . . . he refused, yes. He'd rather die than have it cut off. And he did.[22]

While this example is extreme in magnitude, several widespread procedures have an emotional impact that is often similar in kind. Arthur M. Sutherland, a physician who has written extensively on emotional problems related to cancer, documents the social and emotional consequences of colostomy. According to the psychoanalytic literature, sphincter control is a basic element in socializing the individual. Successful bowel training is the fundamental criterion for social acceptability. Patients who undergo colostomy forfeit much control over their bowel movements, the anatomical structures (rectum, sphincter, and often part of the colon itself) being removed during the surgical procedure. Although patients with a colostomy retain control over their bowel movements to some degree, this control is not nearly as complete as it is among normal individuals. Persons who have undergone colostomies must "irrigate" themselves periodically to clean out their fecal matter with a catheter. This procedure places them in closer contact with their eliminative function than is usual and it is not perfectly reliable. Even persons who follow careful dietary limitations and perform regular irrigation may experience unscheduled bowel movements and spillage of waste material from the stoma.

Sutherland describes several emotional consequences that follow from colostomy. Individuals with colostomies, for example, frequently express feelings of profound self-deprecation, explaining that their bowel activities make them feel "degraded," "debased," "like an animal," and "like a horse."[23] Both male and female patients reported impotency or voluntary discontinuation of sexual activity following this type of surgery. Colostomy also apparently affected the work performance of the men whom Sutherland studied. Of twenty-four men who held jobs before the operation, only seven continued in the same job with no reduced functions, the remaining individuals either dropping out of the labor force, working only sporadically, or accepting positions with significantly less authority and salary than they had enjoyed beforehand. Sutherland reports clear signs of social withdrawal among these individuals, with both men and women restricting their participation in gatherings with relatives and friends, participation at public gatherings, and overnight travel. Sutherland attributes these symptoms of social withdrawal to feelings of physical weakness, inacceptability because of offensive odors and the noise of escaping gas, and the time spent in irrigation. Some patients, he reports, became "veritable recluses because of the colostomy."[24] Of course, colostomy cannot be blamed for the development of all these symptoms. Sutherland comments that patients often used the colostomy as an excuse to cease sexual and work activity and that strong interpersonal relationships and work attachments generally survived problems associated with the surgery.

Many surgical procedures that resemble colostomy in removing organs that play an important part in individual socialization or to which strong emotional feelings are attached have similar social and emotional consequences. Sutherland and his colleagues report that fear of the loss of such organs as a breast, stomach, or uterus may give rise to clinical symptoms including anorexia, insomnia, tachycardia, and emotional manifestations such as indecision, fear, and often panic. Sutherland's studies document that patients frequently connect the prospect of such surgery with feelings of guilt, some, for example, associating hysterectomy with sexual transgressions earlier in life. Case material includes reports of nightmares about "women's breasts hung on meathooks in a butcher shop," regeneration of amputated limbs, and visits from the Angel of Death.[25] Because emotional disturbance is so frequent among patients preceding or following surgery perceived as "mutilating" or identifiable as disruptive to basic character defenses, Sutherland concludes that "patients are at least as concerned with death in surgery or with injury and the probably consequent disruption of their pattern of living" as with dying from cancer.[26] Many widespread though less drastic medical procedures may produce similar though less striking difficulties for emotional adjustment. Hair loss, listlessness, nausea, and other side effects of radiation and chemotherapy may threaten the self-image of many patients and result in their social debilitation. Like the consequences of surgery, these forms of intervention threaten to leave a residue of psychological problems even after physicians have brought the physiological difficulties associated with cancer and its treatment under control.

## MEETING EMOTIONAL NEEDS:
## PROBLEMS FOR THE PROFESSIONAL

If the goal of medical intervention in cancer is to return patients to as normal an approximation of their premorbid states as possible, therapists and planners must take emotional problems as seriously as physical ones. However, the ability of health care professionals and organizations to meet emotional needs related to cancer is highly problematical. Individuals exposed to the emotional needs of patients may lack the personal resources or technical skills necessary to meet them. While the need for effective emotional support is clear, procedures for meeting the need are personally demanding and technically complex. Knowledgeable observers of cancer treatment recommend specific approaches to the problem of assisting emotional adjustment that, if followed, would no doubt improve the lives of numerous patients. Successful performance of this function by a health care organization requires an adequate supply of several distinct resources. Trained and personally confident professionals are, of course, essential. But assigning individuals the responsibility for performing emotional support services in an unambiguous way and assisting them in carrying out these responsibilities is indispensable as well. Organizations can perform no activity in a consistent and effective manner unless they make such specific assignments of responsibility and support individuals so assigned. These "structural" features of task performance are as important in health care as in any other activity and assume particular significance in functions as difficult and complex as providing cancer patients with emotional support.

Providing cancer patients with emotional support is difficult and complex indeed. Whoever assumes the responsibility for the patient's adjustment to cancer and its consequences faces a task that requires time, patience, sensitivity, and emotional strength. The health professional, for example, must begin with a multidimensional evaluation of the patient. How much information is the patient prepared to absorb about the life-threatening condition? How will the possibility of death affect the individual's economic decisions? What effect will his or her demise (or the warning of its approach) have upon family life? What impact will therapeutic intervention have upon the patient's ability to work, recreate, perform family duties, engage in courtship, enjoy sex? Even the most fundamental component of assisting the emotional adjustment of cancer patients requires patient evaluation of the stricken individual's personality, responsibilities, stage in the life cycle, and lastly—perhaps the most evasive of facts to be determined—the individual's wish to know and adjust to the fear-arousing communications.

The task of actually assisting the patient in adjusting to the condition is even more difficult and complex. Again, Sutherland's observations on the psychological problems related to colostomy are highly instructive. He stresses the importance of patient, supportive interaction among patient, family, and health professional. Sutherland identifies the surgeon as "the most important figure in the patient's defenses against anticipation of injury or death."[27] He advises the surgeon to develop a friendly relationship with the patient and to spend time in the preoperative period to insure against the "development of incapacitating beliefs of injury after surgery."[28] He encourages the surgeon to refrain from giving harsh, judgmental, or obscure information, all of which increase the patient's level of anxiety. He cautions those responsible for instructing the patient in irrigation technique against imparting their own negative impression of the procedure, to employ a flexible approach to teaching, and to realize that the inability to learn quickly is not due to willful refusal or dullness, but is related to the "disruptive effects of anxiety and depression."[29] Sutherland's observations on colostomy appear applicable to many other procedures and clinical situations related to cancer. In general, successful emotional adjustment seems to depend on the patient's receiving adequate, nonjudgmental explanations of the condition and procedures for dealing with it, including much encouragement to reconcile himself to the unavoidable consequences of the disease. Aiding the patient's adjustment to cancer, once again, seems to require a working through newly discovered knowledge of experiences, wishes, and facts of life.

Many considerations suggest that health professionals encounter great difficulties in meeting the cancer patient's emotional needs. Physicians, for example, may find their normal method of decisionmaking difficult to apply in dealing with the psychological consequences of malignancies. The physician's normal method of decisionmaking, for example, may be considerably more difficult to apply in emotional areas related to cancer. The complex and painstaking nature of assessing the patient's emotional adjustment parallels the clinical nature of the physician's work. Just as no two patients are exactly alike in the physical sense, no two individuals are identical psychologically. Just as the physician must consider numerous biological facts in deciding how to manage organic illness, the physician must also examine disparate characteristics such as emotional strength, responsibility, and stage in the life cycle and form a unique judgment about each patient. The medical literature on emotional questions related to cancer, in fact, generally suggests that physicians understand the value of the clinical approach to the emotional management of cancer patients.

Observers of health care professionals, though, must question whether the same detached logic that governs conventional medical decisionmaking is generally applied to the emotional aspects of cancer. McIntosh, for example, suggests that fixed ideas about the proper approach to emotional management prevail in the medical profession instead of the willingness to adjust the approach to the unique needs of each patient. About informing patients of the nature of their illness, he comments:

> . . . in a situation of uncertainty about patient responses doctors tend to opt for one extreme or the other with the majority believing in and practicing the ruling that patients should not be told that they have cancer.[30]

The Oken study conveys a similar impression about the enlightenment of cancer patients. Oken remarks:

> More detailed exploration in the interviews cast a great deal of further doubt on the role of experience. It was the exception that a physician could report known examples of the unfavorable consequences of an approach which differed from his own. . . . Instead of logic and rational decision based on clinical observation, what is found is opinion, belief, and conviction, heavily weighted with emotional justification. . . . It would appear that personal conviction is the decisive factor.[31]

Oken concludes that only a minority of the physicians he surveyed tended to be generally flexible in this key area of emotional management of cancer patients.[32]

Personal difficulties compound the technical problems that health professionals face in promoting emotional adjustment among cancer patients. The personal strength required to deal with gravely ill and dying patients is not shared by all health professionals. The briefest exposure of a young health professional to cancer sufferers makes this person well aware of the difficulties involved in emotional contact with them. The prospect of having to face depressed, anxious, or angry patients may deter the health care worker from communicating diagnoses of cancer to them. The necessity of interacting with nasty, unhappy people seems likely to motivate doctors and nurses to adopt stances quite different from the patience and understanding necessary for helping cancer patients adjust to changed body functioning after surgery or other therapeutic procedures. Health professionals unprepared emotionally for these duties seem likely to seek ways to avoid them. The emphasis that professional training programs place upon science (and deemphasis on exposing trainees to emotional trauma facing older individuals) facilitates the avoidance process. In an analysis of medical education and practice, Davis concluded that the doctor's tendency to avoid informing patients of their illness and helping them deal with the disturbing information "is closely related to the practitioner's ability to remove himself from the technically secondary (i.e., nonorganic) problems and issues that follow in the wake of serious illness."[33]

Similar features of the nurses' socialization and technical background may weaken their ability to deal effectively with the cancer patient's emotional needs. As noted in Chapter 5, nursing practice contains an increasingly pervasive scientific component. Although nursing has classically stressed the emotive and nurturing side of care for the ill, today's nursing curricula place stronger emphasis on biomedical material. As among the physicians, nurses may adopt an attitude of avoidance toward the emotional problems of the seriously ill, legitimating such behavior in terms of the newly acquired emphasis in their field. Even more than physicians, nurses may find the demands of the cancer patients burdensome. Nurses are more frequently exposed to direct patient contact and usually render a more intimate variety of services. Added to the emotional needs of the nurse's family, frequent requests for emotional support from patients may motivate the nurse to avoid the time-consuming and personally involving tasks that seem to be necessary to promote adjustments among cancer sufferers.

## PERFORMING THE SUPPORT ROLE: INDIVIDUAL CONTRIBUTIONS AND CONCERN

For many reasons, providing emotional support to cancer patients is as difficult as it is important. A very encouraging feature of our study of the cancer control program, however, was the discovery that many individual nurses and physicians in the Central City region possessed both skill and concern in aiding the emotional adjustment process. A brief review of some of our conversations with these practitioners demonstrates several concrete approaches and procedures that these outstanding individuals were able to integrate into conventional medical practice.

A clinical oncologist interviewed in our study projected a particularly solid impression of confidence and ability in helping cancer patients adjust to their illness. He expressed great sensitivity to the psychological problems of cancer patients, noting that there was "an awful lot of psychiatry" involved in his work. He identified special problems in treating young adults with cancer, commenting that these patients were especially resistant to accepting death. "They act as though they could bargain with you for more time," he commented, recalling pleas that went, "But I've still got a lot of things to do," and "I have so much left to work out." But the oncologist noted that other patients seemed to feel ambivalent about life and death, an attitude that necessitated a special sensitivity. He described a particularly striking case to illustrate the complexities with which a health professional must sometimes deal to determine the need for emotional support and meet it effectively:

> One difficult case—difficult, that is in the emotional sense—was a pretty 21-year old girl with Hodgkin's disease. She actually laughed when we told her the diagnosis. Physiologically, the therapy she underwent was quite successful, but the patient seemed unhappy when we informed her that the lesion had cleared up. I talked to her at length about her feelings, and discovered that she had been raped three years earlier. Due to a strict Catholic upbringing, she felt herself to blame for the incident. When we informed her that she had Hodgkin's disease, she viewed the illness as punishment for the sin, and saw expiation in her approaching death. When she learned that she was not going to die, though, she became depressed. No death meant no absolution.

In this case, the physician referred the patient to a psychiatrist. One must wonder whether the emotional consequences of the disease and its cure would have been serious or even debilitating had the patient not been lucky enough to have a physician sufficiently skilled and concerned to anticipate them.

The extraordinary nature of this case led the oncologist to make a psychiatric referral. But he ordinarily dealt with emotional difficulties related to cancer by himself, integrating emotional support with his other medical activities. One activity, for example, that he felt demanded both a medical and an emotional support role was his position as "anchor man" on a team including several different health professionals. Like other modern diseases, the complexity of cancer necessitates the cooperation of several different medical specialists as well as a variety of nonphysician personnel. This is apparently becoming more prevalent in cancer therapy, where the growing emphasis on multimodal procedures (combining surgery, chemotherapy, and radiation therapy) ordinarily requires the participation of at least three physicians in a single case. As the oncologist pointed out, the cancer patients in his care often passed from the hands of the internist, to those of the radiologist, to those of the resident, nurse, and paraprofessional while hospitalized. The patient, he explained, is "sick, scared, and intimidated by the constant cycle of new faces." As a solution, this physician makes a practice of personally introducing the patient to each individual who will be caring for him or her, giving the patient his card, and letting the patient know that he can be reached "day or night" should the need arise. In this way, the oncologist hoped to provide his patients with a feeling that he was personally concerned with their cases and letting them know that he was both accessible and responsible for the team's performance. In the opinion of this practitioner, the anchor person on the health care team had to be willing to do the necessary "handholding" to allay the patient's feelings of fear and anonymity.

The most striking description of the emotional support component of the oncologist's work came in his description of the mixture of medical and psychological activities in the management of terminal illness and its accompanying pain. According to this practitioner, honesty about the prognosis and appropriate use of narcotics form the basis of successful management of cancer in its terminal stage. The mixture of an emotive and strictly medical component in the oncologist's procedure appears clearly in his description:

It is relatively easy to help a person die if you care and know how . . . I begin by being honest about the prognosis . . . I'll say something like, "Mr. Jones, I cannot cure you of this illness. Here's what I can do. I can help you live as normal and comfortable life as possible for as long as possible. I cannot promise that you will live a specific length of time. But I will promise you this: you will not die in pain."

The connection of drugs with a caring attitude became clearer as the oncologist explained:

> Successfully fulfilling this promise is a matter of the right morphine dosage. Most doctors don't know how to use morphine. The proper way to use it is to keep raising dosages until no more pain is felt. If 50 cc every four hours is prescribed and doesn't work, use 50 cc every three hours. The drug must be prescribed by the clock, because the nurse is usually too busy to see if the patient is still in pain. It is the doctor's responsibility to write out orders and check on the patient.

Similar examples of concerned, able nursing personnel came out in the interviews. A nursing oncology specialist at the university medical center seemed to have the same level of concern and competence as the oncologist described above. A specialist in pediatric nursing, this individual regularly administers chemotherapeutic drugs to victims of leukemia and childhood lymphomas in a specialized pediatric oncology facility. Like the oncologist described above, much of this nurse's emotional support work is mixed with purely technical activity related to cancer treatment. The fact that few children possess as realistic a conception of death as the average adult mitigates the emotional impact of this aspect of cancer. But children are more likely to feel intimidated by the procedures used in treating their illness. While the adult may view the intravenous needle as an annoyance promising the only hope of survival, the child views it as simply a painful and even terrifying ordeal. Thus, the administration of chemotherapy must proceed in as nonthreatening a manner as possible. The ability of the nurse oncology specialist to perform this function was apparent by her popularity among the children at the pediatric facility the day the interviewer visited. It was apprent that the nurse's personal skills, along with the opportunity to treat the same children on a continuing basis, did much to mitigate the terror children might otherwise have felt during chemotherapy sessions.

But the nurse oncology specialist's responsibilities and skills in emotional support went well beyond a warm and understanding personality. If the family is an important part of the picture when cancer strikes an adult, it is even more important for childhood cancer. The death of a child in twentieth-century America may be especially devastating to the family because of the greater "social value" that contemporary society accords to the young in comparison to the old.[34] According to the nurse oncology specialist, counseling the pediatric cancer patient's family was a major part of her duty. Once again, an emotionally supportive role seemed to mix well with a strictly medical one. The nurse would instruct the patient's parents in the nature of the child's illness; she would educate them about the disease's probable course; she would explain chemotherapy treatment and indicate what side effects could be expected. But most important, she would be available whenever needed, either personally or by telephone, to answer questions, give advice, or offer sympathy. The emotive element in this procedure was matched by a medical component. The nurse oncology specialist clearly had to make a judgment about whether a fever indicated an infection—possibly necessitating a midnight trip to the hospital—or an expectable consequence of the chemotherapy.

Another nurse who specialized in cancer work reported impressive results in preparing adult patients for death. She described her activities as intimate physical care for the patient as well as emotional support. This nurse, a woman with strong religious convictions, thought it important to confront the approach of death directly and reconcile oneself to it instead of avoiding its mention. As if to emphasize her beliefs, she referred to herself as a "death and dying nurse" or a "cancer nurse" although her official title was "nursing educator." She described an important part of her work as asking patients how they felt about their approaching death, encouraging them to talk about how their lives had been, and serving as a companion. While these tasks seem simple and obvious, she commented, she was often the only person willing and able to perform them. "Not many people, including the doctors and the families, want to be around dying patients," she explained.

The examples cited above represent only a few well-considered emotional support procedures identified in the study and a small percentage of the professional personnel actively concerned with providing effective emotional support in the region. As suggested throughout this book, however, planners must focus their attention not on extraordinarily devoted individuals, but on the features of the health care system which make important services more or less readily available to the public. A detailed inquiry into the organization of the health care team and the thinking of its members specifically related to emotional support for cancer patients provides information on factors immediately affecting the delivery of these services. Information of this kind comes as close as possible to indicating the effects of current patterns of social relations in the health care industry upon actual patient services without utilizing outcome measures, indicators of a type perhaps impossible to obtain in the emotional support area.

## THE RESPONSIBILITY FOR EMOTIONAL ADJUSTMENT

The support that health professionals themselves receive from colleagues and work organizations encourages or discourages them from performing specific tasks and helps or hinders them in performing these tasks effectively. Among the most effective providers of emotional support cited above, feelings of personal responsibility clearly promoted delivery of needed services. Religious convictions played an important part in the motivation of the "death and dying" nurse. Modern health care organizations, however, cannot depend on such externally based factors. Effective control of the emotional effects of cancer requires direct encouragement arising within the health care organization itself for providing patients with the support they need.

Perhaps the most basic question investigators can ask about provision of emotional support in organizations that care for cancer patients concerns allocation of responsibility for the task. The clear designation of particular individuals on the health care team as being responsible for aiding the patient's emotional adjustment is particularly important in insuring that the function is performed. Persons who find themselves in the position to perform a needed function will be encouraged to fulfill that responsibility despite their personal predilections against doing so if they have received specific instructions for the task during professional training or on the job. Individuals who realize a specific patient need but who have received formal or informal word that the responsibility belongs to someone else will feel inhibited from taking action whatever their personal predilections. Because cancer and other serious illnesses are so emotionally charged and socially consequential—with the approach of death, for example, the duties of family members may conflict with those of doctors and nurses—the health professional must have a clear feeling of legitimacy if he or she is to perform the emotional support role comfortably. Thus, the question of whether health professionals unambiguously identify the emotional support role as their legitimate responsibility is a particularly appropriate indicator of whether the health care organizations in the cancer control program service region perform this service reliably and effectively.

The Professional Community Survey included a series of items designed to determine whether specific individuals—physicians, nurses, or relatives—felt a clear responsibility to assist the cancer patient in making an emotional adjustment to the condition. The responses to these questions first provide clues to the presence or absence of persons to whom the cancer patient can turn for emotional support in actual treatment settings. Second, responses to these questions help determine whether the professionals surveyed could identify any single type of individual with both the ability and the responsibility to aid the cancer patient's emotional adjustment. We felt that any health care system that reliably provided for this need would train the occupants of specific roles in meeting the emotional problems of cancer patients and designate which persons should provide this type of care. We reasoned that if the system did, in fact, include such individuals, health care professionals would be able to identify them unambiguously. The absence of even a weak consensus about who should and does play the most important role in helping the cancer patient adjust to the condition, however, would constitute evidence that the health care system included no specific category of personnel who performed this function legitimately and well.

The survey asked respondents to rank the patient's family, the nurse, and the doctor according to their relative importance in helping cancer patients adjust to their illness. The survey first asked who *should* play the most important role and second who *does* play the most important role in the cancer patient's adjustment. Tables 6-1 through 6-6 summarize the results of this questioning.

Tables 6-1 and 6-2 show that physicians and nurses agree in some respects about who should have primary responsibility for the cancer patient's emotional adjustment but disagree in others. Few nurses or physicians, for example, seem to feel that the nurse should play the most important role in the patient's emotional adjustment. Although significantly more nurses than doctors feel that nurses should play the most important role (see Table 6-1), only 7.3 percent of the nurses sampled actually expressed this opinion. Similarly, Table 6-1 shows no significant difference between the percentage of nurses and physicians who think that the family should play the most important role. An important difference in the nurses' and physicians' impression of the proper role of the physician, though, appears in this table. While the majority of physicians questioned think that physicians should play the most important part in patient adjustment, only a minority of the nurses agree. The difference between the percentage of physicians and nurses who think that physicians should play the most important role is statistically significant.

Table 6-2, which indicates which type of individual physicians and nurses think *does* play the most important role in the cancer pa-

Table 6-1.   Who Should Aid the Patient's Emotional Adjustment to Cancer?[a]

| These Professionals: | Physicians | Nurses | $\chi^2$ |
|---|---|---|---|
| Believe that these parties should play the most important part: | | | |
| Physicians | 50.6 (42) | 28.1 (27) | 8.57[b] |
| Nurses | 0 | 7.3 (7) | 4.44[c] |
| Family | 41.0 (34) | 51.0 (49) | 1.44 |

[a]Percentages in this table have been abstracted from three fourfold tables ($df$ = 1) cross-tabulating occupational specialty with belief that physicians, nurses, or family should play the most important role. Numbers in parentheses represent number in each occupational category who think that specified party should play the most important role.
[b]$p < .01$.
[c]$p < .05$.

Table 6-2.   Who Actually Plays the Most Important Part in Aiding the Patient's Emotional Adjustment?[a]

| These Professionals: | Physicians | Nurses | $\chi^2$ |
|---|---|---|---|
| Believe that these parties do play the most important part:   — | | | |
| Physicians | 54.4 (43) | 12.8 (12) | 32.47[b] |
| Nurses | 2.6 (2) | 43.2 (41) | 35.18[b] |
| Family | 33.3 (26) | 27.7 (26) | 0.41 |

[a]Percentages in this table have been abstracted from three fourfold tables ($df$ = 1) cross-tabulating occupational specialty with belief that physicians, nurses, or family do play the most important role. Numbers in parentheses represent number in each occupational category who think that specified party does play the most important role.
[b]$p < .01$.

tient's emotional adjustment, implies even more disagreement. While similar percentages of nurses and physicians agree that the family *does* play the most important role, dissension prevails in their evaluation of others who may perform the function. While over 54 percent of the physicians questioned, for example, feel that they and members of their profession do play the most important role, only a small minority of the nurses agree. The differences in the percentages of doctors and nurses who think that physicians play the most important role is significant at the 0.01 level. Nurses, furthermore, think that they *do* play the most important role in patient adjustment far more frequently than doctors attribute this role to them. Over 43 percent of the nurses questioned believe that they play the most important role, compared with slightly over 2 percent of the physicians. The difference is significant at the 0.01 level.

According to Tables 6-1 and 6-2, physicians and nurses express different evaluations of the roles each plays in emotional support for patients. Physicians and nurses differ most strikingly in their estimation of the physician's proper role. Nurses think that doctors both should and do play a less important role in the patient's emotional adjustment than the doctors themselves think. Nurses also feel that members of *their* profession play a more important role in assisting the patient's adjustment than the physicians are willing to attribute to them.

The question of whether physicians and nurses think they themselves play appropriate roles in providing cancer patients with emotional support is also important in helping determine whether the health care system (or the small part of it examined in this study) successfully assigns particular individuals with the task of performing this function. Tables 6-3 through 6-5 shed considerable light on this issue. As Table 6-3 indicates, most physicians who feel they should play the most important role in helping the cancer patient adjust to the condition also feel they *do*, in fact, play this role; the vast majority of physicians who feel they should not play the most important

Table 6-3. The Physician's Perception of His or Her Role in Aiding Patient's Adjustment[a]

| | | Physician *should* play most important role in patient's adjustment | |
| | | Yes | No |
|---|---|---|---|
| Physician *does* play most important role in patient's adjustment | Yes | 82.1 [40.5][a] | 27.5 [13.9] |
| | No | 17.9 [ 8.9] | 72.5 [36.7] |
| | 100% = | (39) | (40) |

$\chi^2$ = 21.54, $p < .001$, gamma = 0.85.

[a]Figures in brackets represent percentage of all physicians included in each cell of the table.

role report that they do not, in fact, do so. Physicians, therefore, usually feel they act as they should in the emotional support area.

In some respects, nurses follow a pattern similar to the physicians. As Table 6-4 indicates, a majority of the nurses who thought they should play the most important role in aiding the patient's emotional adjustment reported that they did, in fact, perform this function. Like the physicians, the majority of nurses who thought they should not play the most important role expressed the feeling that they, in fact, did not. However, the perceptions of nurses and physicians differ in an important respect; a sizable minority of the nurses sampled feel they do play the most important role in aiding the patient's adjustment but, in fact, should not. Almost 38 percent of the nurses sampled fell into this category, compared with under 14 percent of the physicians (see Table 6-3). While the majority of physicians and nurses felt they played the appropriate role in the emotional support area, then, a nonnegligible percentage of the nurses reported performing a function they felt they should not perform. The comparison of the physicians' and nurses' perceptions of appropriateness of their roles in the emotional support area appears in Table 6-5. This table shows that a significantly higher percentage of the physicians sampled interpreted the role they played in helping the cancer patient adapt to the condition as appropriate for their profession.

Thus, a degree of ambivalence appears in the health professionals' perceptions about who does and should take primary responsibility for assisting the patient's emotional adjustment. Physicians generally

Table 6-4.  The Nurse's Perception of His or Her Role in Aiding Patient's Adjustment[a]

|  |  | Nurse *should* play most important role in patient's adjustment | |
| --- | --- | --- | --- |
|  |  | *Yes* | *No* |
| Nurse *does* play most important role in patient's adjustment | *Yes* | 71.4 [ 5.3][a] | 40.9 [37.9] |
|  | *No* | 28.6 [ 2.1] | 59.1 [54.7] |
|  | 100% = | (7) | (88) |

$\chi^2$ = 1.38, $p$ = n.s., gamma = 0.57.

[a]Figures in brackets represent percentage of all nurses included in each cell of the table.

Table 6-5. Percentage in Each Occupational Specialty Who Feel They Play Appropriate Role in Patient's Adjustment

|  |  | Occupational Specialty | |
|  |  | *Physician* | *Nurse* |
| Plays appropriate role | *Yes* | 76.6 | 60.0 |
|  | *No* | 23.4 | 40.0 |
|  | 100% = | (77) | (95) |

$\chi^2 = 4.62, p < .05$, gamma = 0.37.

think they should and do perform this role, and the minority of doctors who report not playing the most important role feel they should not play it. Nurses, though, often feel they do play the most important role but should not.

It is useful to think of the data reported in Tables 6-1 through 6-5 as aggregates of observations rather than attitudes. The nurses and physicians sampled here, after all, spend a good deal of time both caring for people with cancer and observing the activities of others in the same role. The degree of discensus that appears in their evaluations of each other suggests that there is no particular professional to whom the patient may always look for emotional support. Rather, some professionals think of themselves as performing the most important function in this area, while others estimate the value of their efforts well below this level. Some individuals think they perform the most important role but feel somehow they are not the appropriate ones to take care of this activity. Many doctors and nurses individually perform valuable services in emotional support. But it seems quite likely that numerous physicians perform a less effective role than they think (this is why the nurses often say they should not play the most important role) and that nurses frequently feel inhibited from aiding the patient either because they do not consider it within their proper domain or receive criticism from the physicians for offering the service.

If the nurses and physicians sampled in this study are accurate observers of the parts of the health care system that treat cancer patients in the Central City region, many patients may find little emotional support among the professionals they encounter. Cancer patients whose health care team includes physicians who perform emotional support services ineffectively *and* whose nurses feel inhibited from attempting to deliver the service may find no professional able to give them the help they need. Emotional support services may be unavailable because of the inability of the health care organization to provide able individuals with the feeling that they may legitimately play the support role.

The possibility that no specific professional in a given health care setting may offer skillful emotional support with the backing of other health professionals is particularly serious in the light of the findings reported in Table 6-6. This table indicates that relatively few of the physicians and nurses questioned feel that the patient's family both should and does play the most important role in promoting emotional adjustment. Fewer than a quarter of those questioned felt that the family both did and should play this role. In contrast, nearly a majority of the nurses and physicians (45.9 percent) felt that the family neither should nor did play the major part in patient adjustment, while a large number of respondents (23.8 percent) indicated that although the family should play the major role, it did not. Perhaps these impressions of the role the family does and should play stem from observations by nurses and physicians of unsuccessful attempts by families to aid their sick and dying kin. Perhaps many of these professionals feel families should play this role but avoid responsibility of doing so. In either case, the respondents to the Professional Community Survey often feel emotional support is not a job for the family. If these professionals are indeed accurate observers, Table 6-6 has disturbing implications; the omissions of the health care system in the emotional support area are not filled by the traditional source of emotional support in other areas, the family.

The impression that neither doctors, nurses, nor family can be

Table 6-6. Perception Among Physicians and Nurses of Family's Role in Aiding Patient's Adjustment

|  |  | Family *should* play most important role | |
|  |  | Yes | No |
| Family *does* play most important role | Yes | 49.4 [23.3]a | 13.2 [ 7.0] |
|  | No | 50.6 [23.8] | 86.8 [45.9] |
|  | 100% = | (81) | (91) |

$\chi^2$ = 24.9, $p <$ .001, gamma = 0.73.

aFigures in brackets represent percentage of all physicians and nurses included in each cell of the table.

counted upon to provide emotional support was echoed by an experienced oncologist. Commenting on the findings from the Professional Community Survey, this physician said that, in his experience, hospital porters and janitors played the major role in providing cancer patients with emotional support. These persons appeared in the hospital room after doctors, nurses, and family had all departed, and, unconstrained by personal or professional inhibitions provided patients with conversation, sympathy, and comfort when they were needed most.

## A WORKING HYPOTHESIS

The data presented in Tables 6-1 through 6-5 suggest that many persons within the health professions either feel they should not perform the emotional support roles they do or that others who perform these roles do so inadequately. Although particular *individuals* clearly respond effectively to the emotional needs of cancer patients, the health care system does not seem to assign any particular role the responsibility for this important activity. As suggested above, this may result in the absence of emotional support for patients without adequate family and friendship resources for this. What factors prevent the health care system from developing responsibilities vested in particular roles—be they in medicine, nursing, or some other category of health care worker—for emotional support of cancer patients, responsibilities that are regarded as legitimate by all and are carried out effectively?

As a working hypothesis, it seems likely that several factors have combined to produce a systemic neglect within the health care system of emotional support for cancer patients. First, physicians often appear to feel that their role as chief executive of the health care team gives them the primary responsibility for emotional support. Yet many constraints keep them from adequately carrying out the responsibility. Most important among these are (1) lack of time, (2) lack of adequate preparation, and (3) lack of sufficient personal confidence to carry out the task. Even when one or a combination of these factors prevents the doctor from performing effectively as an agent of emotional support, however, many practitioners retain the feeling that they in fact do meet their responsibilities in this area by (1) developing an illusory conception that they in fact perform the task or (2) minimizing the importance of the cancer patient's emotional problems. Nurses, for their part, are unwilling to share the illusion held by many physicians that they fulfill whatever emotional needs the patient has and, hence, report the impression that physicians in fact do not play the most important part in the cancer patient's emotional adjustment. Instead, many nurses feel that *they* play the most important part, but seldom feel they should do the job. The ineffectiveness of the physicians, they seem to think, leaves them with a responsibility they are unable to fulfill for the following reasons: (1) they lack sufficient training to perform the role as well as they should; (2) they lack sufficient professional discretion on the health care team to fulfill the responsibility; and (3) they, like the physicians, often lack the required level of personal confidence and emotional preparation.

These factors are numerous and complex. Differing combinations of these factors may condition the attitudes and performance of professionals differently in specific organizations and localities. But the *individual* factors suggested above are quite likely to be present everywhere in the contemporary health care system, and they merit thorough exploration.

### Time

Among the most important factors that condition the ability of health professionals to provide effective emotional support for the cancer patient is the *time* they have for performing the task. Modern medicine, of course, stresses the importance of concrete, scientifically based techniques, aimed at the physiological problems of the patient. The principal time demands facing the physician fall into this area. It is certain that many physicians who would *like* to provide emotional support for their patients simply do not have time in view of the strictly technical task they are required to carry out.

Several central features of modern hospital-based practice exaggerate the time constraints that face even physicians strongly motivated to assist their patients in making an emotional adjustment to cancer. The average physician, for example, spends only a small proportion of time in the hospital, devoting the bulk of the working hours to office practice and, if he or she has an academic connection, to research and teaching. The hours spent in the hospital must be divided among numerous patients, perhaps allowing only a few moments for each. Therefore, physicians seldom have the time to engage in the working through of information and determining the patient's ability to cope that Sutherland and others have identified as critical parts of cancer treatment.

Other health professionals, of course, spend more time in the hospital and have more face-to-face contact with cancer patients in this setting. The residents on the hospital house staff, for example, spend essentially all their time in the hospital and are more exposed to the patient. The same is true of nurses and other nonphysician health care workers. But the time constraints on these personnel are also great, emphasizing activities other than emotional support. Like other young professionals, residents are essentially apprentices in the medical community. As such, they tend to receive assignments of standardized procedures and technical details that attending physicians prefer to avoid. Thus, the resident is often too busy to devote much attention to the patient's emotional needs. The same is true of the majority of nurses. These professionals also perform standardized duties, often finding themselves unable to break out of the cycle of routine procedures long enough to provide conversation and sympathy.

### Preparation

The Professional Community Survey generates evidence that a relatively small number of medical professionals receive sufficient preparation to meet the emotional needs of cancer patients. A series of items on the survey questionnaire asked respondents to rate the quality of the preparation they received both in professional school and postgraduate experience to meet both the psychological and physiological needs of cancer patients. Tables 6-7 and 6-8, which present the outcomes of this series of questions, provide an indication of the ability of the present educational system to prepare medical professionals for the task of assisting emotional adjustment.

A comparison of the quality health professionals associate with their preparation to meet the psychological and physiological needs of cancer patients is especially instructive. In general, the professionals responding to the survey seem to feel that their preparation to meet the physical needs of cancer patients is superior to their training in the illness's emotional side. Table 6-7 indicates, for example, that 23.5 percent of the physicians and 38.9 percent of the nurses surveyed felt their training in professional school to meet the emotional needs of cancer patients was very good to excellent. In comparison, Table 5-8 shows that 47.6 percent of the physicians and 55.3 percent of the nurses felt that their preparation to meet the physiological needs of cancer patients was very good to excellent. By a statistically significant margin ($p < .05$) both nurses and physicians felt that their preparation to meet the physiological needs of cancer patients was more frequently very good to excellent than their training in meeting the patient's psychological needs.

Training outside the classroom is, of course, more important to many aspects of health care than instruction in professional school. The physician is likely to learn anatomy, physiology, and biochemis-

Table 6-7.   Percentages of Physicians and Nurses Who Perceive the Quality of Their Preparation to Meet the Psychological Needs of Cancer Patients as Very Good to Excellent[a]

|  | *Occupational Specialty* | | |
| --- | --- | --- | --- |
|  | *Physicians* | *Nurses* | $\chi^2$ |
| Preparation in professional school | 23.5 (19) | 38.9 (37) | 4.15[b] |
| Postgraduate experience | 56.8 (46) | 44.4 (36) | 2.00 |

[a]Percentages in table abstracted from two fourfold tables ($df = 1$). Figures in parentheses represent numbers in each occupational category who consider their preparation in professional school or postgraduate experience very good to excellent.
[b]$p < .05$.

Table 6-8.   Percentage of Physicians and Nurses Who Perceive the Quality of Their Preparation to Meet Physical Needs of Cancer Patients as Very Good to Excellent[a]

|  | *Occupational Specialty* | | |
| --- | --- | --- | --- |
|  | *Physicians* | *Nurses* | $\chi^2$ |
| Preparation in professional school | 47.6 (39) | 55.3 (52) | 0.77 |
| Postgraduate experience | 75.5 (62) | 58.0 (47) | 5.50[b] |

[a]Percentages in table abstracted from two fourfold tables ($df = 1$). Figures in parentheses represent numbers in each occupational category who consider their preparation in professional school or postgraduate experience very good to excellent.
[b]$p < .05$.

try in the classroom, but suturing, dressing, and drug dosages are learned on the wards during residency. Postgraduate training, then, is more important to the physician in developing practical skills in patient care. To some degree, the same seems true of nurses during their early years on the wards. According to Tables 6-7 and 6-8, both physicians and nurses report the impression that their preparation to meet the physiological needs of cancer patients is more frequently very good to excellent than their preparation in the emotional area. Again, the differences in percentages who feel their postgraduate preparation of this calibre in the physiological area (75.5 percent for doctors and 58.0 percent for nurses) is significantly greater than in the emotional area (56.8 percent for doctors, 44.4 percent for nurses). The differences for both nurses and physicians are significant at the .05 level.

Table 6-7 suggests that relatively few health professionals feel highly qualified to meet the emotional needs of cancer patients. Only a minority of the nurses surveyed feel that their training was very good to excellent in this area, whether acquired in professional school or postgraduate experience. A bare majority of physicians feel that their training in meeting the cancer patient's emotional needs during postgraduate training was very good to excellent. But the observer must interpret this statistic with a degree of qualification. First, the observer must recall that much of the postgraduate training of the physician aims at developing "clinical judgment," a variety of expertise whose consistency is difficult to evaluate and, according to several analysts already cited, frequently exaggerated in value. Second, the physician may underestimate the magnitude of the emotional support role, consequently overestimating the adequacy of his or her preparation to play the role successfully.

Table 6-9 provides some useful perspectives on this question. The table summarizes responses to a series of items specifically aimed at determining the way professionals perceived the cancer patient's emotional needs. The first item appearing in the table asked respondents whether most people with cancer whom they cared for were "adequately prepared to deal with it." This item was intended to

**Table 6-9. Attitudes Toward Patient Care Among Physicians and Nurses (Percentages Agreeing Within Each Occupational Specialty)[a]**

|  | *Occupational Specialty* | | |
| --- | --- | --- | --- |
|  | *Physician* | *Nurse* | $\chi^2$ |
| (1) Cancer patients are prepared to cope | 34.9 (29) | 16.0 (15) | 7.52[b] |
| (2) Cancer patients are difficult to talk with | 26.5 (22) | 53.7 (51) | 12.43[b] |
| (3) Patients prefer not to know about their conditions | 41.0 (32) | 25.3 (24) | 4.17[c] |

[a]Percentages in table have been abstracted from three fourfold tables ($df$ =1) cross-tabulating occupational specialty and agreement with each attitude item. Numbers in parentheses represent numbers in each occupational category who say they agree or agree strongly with specified item.
[b]$p < .01$.
[c]$p < .05$.

help determine the respondent's overall estimation of the patient's emotional resources in dealing with the disease. The next item, asking respondents whether they felt most cancer patients with whom they dealt "were difficult to talk with about their condition," aimed at determining the professional's own estimation of one important emotional support activity, that of communication. The final item, asking whether cancer patients "would prefer not to know too much about their condition, even though they say otherwise," was designed to determine the respondent's impression about the need to inform patients about the facts of their cases.

The differences in responses to this series of questions by physicians and nurses suggest vast differences in perceptions of the patient's emotional needs. It would appear that physicians estimate these needs consistently lower than nurses. Nurses, for example, are only about half as likely as physicians to feel that cancer patients are adequately prepared to cope with their illness. The difference in the percentage of nurses and physicians who agree with this statement is significant at the .01 level. Nurses, furthermore, consider it difficult to talk with cancer patients about their condition about twice as often as physicians. Again, the difference is significant at the .01 level. Finally, a significantly higher percentage of the physicians surveyed ($p < .05$) felt that cancer patients preferred not to know about their condition.

As suggested above, interpretation of these data must remain guarded. The data in Table 6-9, though, are entirely consistent with the hypothesis that physicians underestimate the emotional problems of cancer patients in many instances. Clearly, the physician sees each of the problem areas reflected in the items in Table 6-9 as less serious than the nurse. Given this lower estimation of the magnitude of the problem, it is easy to see why physicians may feel their preparation is more adequate than the nurse even if the absolute values of the training received by both classes of professions were essentially the same.

### Personal Confidence

In addition to such concrete factors as lack of time and insufficient preparation in the technical sense for providing emotional support for cancer patients, indications arose in the study of personnel at the university medical center of strictly personal factors affecting the ability of individuals to perform this function. Many aspects of cancer are, of course, frightening not only to victims of the disease but also to others around them. Apparently, the psychologically threatening features of cancer are as disturbing to health professionals as to lay people.

The observations of a psychiatrist closely connected with the cancer control program suggested several reasons why physicians, nurses, and other health professionals either felt uncomfortable in the emotional support role or performed the function poorly. The psychiatrist suggested that many physicians thought of cancer as a personal threat, first, because they could not cure many of its forms and, second, because it symbolized their own mortality. "The implied threat on the physician's mortality inhibits the development of a positive relationship with cancer patients," the psychiatrist commented. The medical literature suggests similar connections between physicians' personal background and attitudes and their ability to form emotionally supportive relationships with cancer patients. Easson writes that in treating cancer patients the physician's response to the possibility of treatment failure or death

> . . . is determined by uniquely personal beliefs, emotions, and experiences. His philosophy about his own death may be subtly interwoven with his attitudes towards others. . . . Conventional medical education has done little to equip the young doctor with knowledge of how to convey a diagnosis of a potentially fatal disease, or how to offer continuing emotional support along with physical care.[35]

These observations would doubtlessly be equally accurate for many nurses and other health professionals who come into contact with cancer patients.

The tendency of individuals in any occupation or stage of the life cycle to experience problems in retaining emotional contact with seriously ill and dying people is understandable. The problematical element in this picture, though, is whether those who enter the health professions could be more effectively prepared and organized to provide this support. In providing a tentative model to explain why the health care system does not specify a particular, unambiguously designated set of individuals to perform the emotional support function, the factors presented above suggest both a solution to the problem and difficulties in putting the solution into effect.

## A TENTATIVE CONCLUSION

Lack of time, training, and emotional preparation for aiding the emotional adjustment of cancer patients to their condition seems to accompany the ambivalence that many doctors and nurses project in their interpretation of how this function is performed. These three factors all appear to affect both nurses and physicians, limiting their ability to provide emotional support for cancer patients. But the direct influence of these factors on the thoughts and actions of the health professionals sampled in this study does not explain why physicians and nurses feel differently about the roles each plays in the emotional support area. Why, for example, should the majority of physicians feel they play the most important role in aiding patient adjustment while only a tiny minority of nurses agree that they in fact play this role (see Table 6-2)? Why should a significant minority of nurses indicate they play the most important role, but feel they should not (Table 6-4)? Based on the explanations of several health professionals participating in the study, the factors of time, training, and emotional preparation affect nurses and physicians differently. The difference between the responses of each professional specialty to difficulties related to emotional support for cancer patients highlights major problems planners and other innovators can expect to encounter in seeing that this function is performed more reliably.

Physicians seem to respond to the problems faced in providing emotional support by distancing themselves from the patient. By either limiting their contact with the patient or pretending that the emotional problems related to cancer are smaller than they actually are, physicians remove themselves from feeling responsible for providing a type of care that they feel unable to deliver. Physicians can do many things that allow them to retain the impression that they are performing more of the emotional support task than is actually the case. They can act cheerful around the patient whose real needs are for someone to sympathize with the gravity of his or her condition. They can physically absent themselves from the patient's company. They can declare to other members of the health care team that they and they alone will provide all the information, communication, and empathy that the patient needs. In this way, doctors may feel that they are doing the required job and explicitly or implicitly enjoin other health care workers from competing for the role. This distancing strategy, though, produces much of the ambivalence toward the emotional support function that this chapter reports. The absenting strategy of physicians lets them think they play the major support role, but it leads the nurse to express the opinion that they do not play this role at all.

Nurses, on the other hand, remain in contact with the patient after the doctor has physically or emotionally departed. Because they enjoy less flexibility in their work than doctors (continuing to perform intimate patient care in a routine manner), the patient is likely to press the *nurse* for information, empathy, and other components of human interaction required to promote emotional adjustment. As detailed in Chapter 5, some of the central values of the nursing profession make the opportunity to provide emotional support in the doctor's absence quite attractive. It seems likely, though, that the nurse as an individual feels as little prepared (technically or emotionally) as the physician and retains the implied or stated warning from the physician not to encroach on a function the physician defines as his or her own. For this reason, nurses feel they *should not* provide the patient's major component of emotional support, even when they feel they somehow end up doing so.

Evidence to support this conclusion appeared throughout the study. The tendency of physicians to identify the presence of difficult emotional problems among cancer patients with considerably less frequency than nurses (Table 6-9) provides indirect support for this conclusion. Data from interviews with nurses and physicians in the cancer control program service region provide support of a more direct nature. The comments of the psychiatrist quoted earlier are especially instructive. He described the development of medical practice in the late twentieth century as an attempt of physicians to remove themselves father and farther from the more disagreeable aspects of patient care. He explained:

> Much of the public thinks that the physician's work involves regular exposure to revolting features of caring for sick people. Outsiders see medicine as a profession which is well paid, but requires contact with screaming patients, bad smells, blood, vomitus, and feces. This is not really true. Doctors today have placed many other individuals between themselves and all these disagreeable features of care for the sick. The physician doesn't clean up the vomit, that's the orderly's job. The doctor doesn't have to stick needles into patients, the nurses or maybe the residents do that. Now a whole new category of paraprofessionals is emerging which will allow physicians to remain even farther from the patient.
>
> Doctors are especially anxious to place other people between themselves and cancer patients. The cancer patient, especially in the terminal stage, often needs sympathy, reassurance, or just plain companionship. The physician is not trained to provide this support. Medical schools don't teach students how important it is. Most physicians do not have the emotional orientation necessary to provide it. We are trained to be stoics, to detach ourselves from the "emotionalism" of patients. So many of us turn our backs on the problem. The average doctor only spends two or three hours in the hospital per week, anyway. We leave the nurses to handle the situation, whether they are prepared for it or not.

Other studies of the health professional's treatment of cancer patients have documented similar mechanisms by which physicians avoid playing the emotional support role, leaving it to others by default. In the matter of enlightening patients about their diagnosis, Glaser and Strauss note that "because doctors in general choose not to inform cancer patients about their condition, the burden of coping with the patients falls fairly and squarely on the shoulders of the nurses."[36] Similarly, McIntosh writes that "As doctors tend not to be very forthcoming in giving information to cancer patients, it is likely that the patient will be thrown towards other members of the staff, such as nurses and social workers in order to find out about their condition."[37]

Even among the nurses in the present study who recognized the importance of filling the vacancy in the emotional support area, actual performance of the function seemed to take place in an inhibited and often surreptitious manner. One nurse, for example, reported that she made a practice of hinting strongly to a patient that he or she had cancer, the resulting enlightenment enabling her to discuss the patient's condition with him or her in a reasonably uninhibited way. Others, though, suggested that nursing personnel were just as anxious to avoid these emotionally taxing roles as the doctors. Established boundaries of responsibility and the scientific component of the value system in nursing facilitatate *their* avoidance. As still another study of professionals and cancer patients concludes:

> This professional rationale also serves an important self-protective function since the nurse can legitimately avoid seeking out information (and responsibilities) which is not essential for the successful performance of her job. . . . Avoidance maneuvers protect the self image of the nurse as a saver of lives but also prevent strong feelings and fears about death from being brought to the surface.[38]

Both the data collected in the study of Central City University's Cancer Control Program and judgments arising from other research suggest a discouraging conclusion about the ability of the contemporary health care system to help the cancer patient adjust emotionally to the condition. No role within the health professions appears to include a trained capacity and a universally supported assignment to perform the function. A reasonable though unhappy conclusion is that many cancer patients simply do not receive any effective assistance in making an adjustment to their condition. This omission may result in concrete impairment of life among those who are cured and, for those who must die, deaths significantly more horrifying than they need to be. This conclusion is stated as "tentatate" merely because the data presented here include no direct observation of emotional support activity. The indirect approach taken here, though, has the advantage of combining the observations of many independent observers. The resulting numerical data add weight to previous studies based on direct observation. The conclusions of both this and other studies argue strongly for arrangements that improve the capacity of the health care system to provide emotional support for the seriously ill.

Designating a particular type of health professional to perform the emotional support role might possibly improve the capacity of the health care system to provide emotional support to those who lacked friends and family capable of performing the service. The vesting of responsibility for this function in a specific occupational role would eliminate much of the confusion about who should perform the task that prevails at present. The nursing profession seems to be the most logical place to vest specific responsibility for the emotional support role. As discussed in Chapter 5, the professional values of nurses seem to retain much more of the nutritive and empathetic aspect of health care than those of physicians. Given these proclivities within nursing, it seems highly possible to select a sufficient number of nurses for special training in emotional support for cancer patients. The elements of the cancer control program educational outreach effort that offered nurses further training in the emotional needs of cancer patients were important preliminary steps in this direction.

In view of the structural characteristics of the contemporary health care system, though, this solution has an extremely naive quality. The same factors that discourage nurses from comfortably assuming the emotional support role on an informal basis at present may cripple future attempts to formally allocate the function to them. Recall, for example, that nurses responding to the Professional Community Survey typically take a passive attitude toward patient care in their relation with physicians. Chapter 5 indicates that only a minority of nurses regularly initiate contact with physicians about specific persons with cancer and that only a minute fraction of the physicians report being asked frequently by nurses to see specific cancer patients. These responses suggest that basic changes in the authority system surrounding cancer treatment will have to take place before the nurse can perform an expanded emotional support role reliably and effectively. If the current authority system remains intact, special selection and training of nurses may represent a gross waste of resources and result in higher expectations among the nursing labor force that will remain unmet. Physicians, for example, may choose to retain their control over the flow of information on diagnoses. Without being encouraged to participate in the decision to enlighten cancer patients about their condition, it is difficult to see how the nurse could adopt the open and direct stance necessary to provide effective emotional support. In extreme cases, physicians may simply direct the nurse to refrain from discussing the patients' condition with them, despite special training the nurse may have received in this field.

Patterns of authority governing the relations of doctors and nurses, though, are only one feature of the present social technology in health care that reduces the system's ability to control cancer more effectively. Other features of this social technology include a system of medical education that places decreasing emphasis on the emotional side of illness, a value system among physicians that places low priority on activities related to emotional support, and a reward system in health care that provides handsome fees for the performance of concrete medical procedures, but offers little tangible reward for communication and reassurance of seriously ill patients. Improved cancer control depends on alterations in the relations among health professionals and the priorities of the health care system as well as new educational offerings.

This book has suggested several ways in which the social technology currently used by the health care system affects the behavior of specific health professionals and, in turn, limits their ability to advance the goals of cancer control. It has dealt thus far with only one actual service affected by the system's operations, emotional support for cancer patients. Chapter 7 addresses another important service in the health care system's array of cancer-fighting activities. While it considers elements of the social technology similar to those discussed here—interpersonal relations within health care organizations—it also includes a perspective on integration among the separate organizational units composing the health care system as a whole.

## NOTES

1. B. Cobb, "Why Do People Detour to Quacks?" *Psychiatric Bulletin* 4 (1954): 66-69.

2. J.E. Holland and E. Frei III, *Cancer Medicine* (Philadelphia: Lea and Febiger, 1973).

3. J. McIntosh, *Communication and Awareness in a Cancer Ward* (New York: Prodist, 1977), p. 59.

4. Ibid., p. 64.

5. Ibid., p. 65.

6. W.T. Fitts and I.S. Raudin, "What Philadelphia Physicians Tell Patients with Cancer," *Journal of the American Medical Association* 153 (1953), p. 901.

7. D. Rennick, "What Should Physicians Tell the Cancer Patient," *New Medica Materia* 2 (March, 1960): 51-53.

8. D. Oken, "What to Tell Cancer Patients," *Journal of the American Medical Association* 86 (1961). See p. 1126.

9. F. Davis, "Uncertainty in Medical Prognosis, Clinical and Functional," *Medical Care*, W.R. Scott and E.H. Volkart, eds. (New York: John Wiley, 1966). See p. 319.

10. *Canterbury* v. *Spence*, 464 F.2d 772 (1972).

11. McIntosh, op. cit., p. 193.

12. Ibid., p. 199

13. Ibid., p. 174

14. A. Gerlert et al., "The Patient with Inoperable Cancer from the Psychiatric and Social Standpoints," *Cancer* 13 (1960), p. 1206.

15. M.J. Krant, M. Beiser, G. Adler, and L. Johnston, "The Role of a Hospital-Based Psychosocial Unit in Terminal Cancer Illness and Bereavement," *Journal of Chronic Disease* 29 (1976): 115-127. See pp. 118-119.

16. McIntosh, op. cit., Chapter 10.

17. A. Peck, "Emotional Reactions to Having Cancer," *American Journal Roent, Radiol and Nuclear Medicine* 114 (1972): 591-599.

18. E. Freidson, *Professional Dominance: The Social Structure of Medical Care* (New York: Atherton Press, 1970). See p. 86.

19. A.C. Ernstene, "Explaining to the Patient: A Professional Tool and a Professional Obligation," *Journal of the American Medical Association* 165 (1972): 165.

20. R. Moses and C. Nizze, "Differential Levels of Awareness of Illness: Their Relation to Some Salient Features of Cancer Patients," *New York Academy of Science* 21 (January, 1966): 984-994.

21. Peck, op. cit., pp. 591-599.

22. McIntosh, op. cit., p. 70.

23. A.M. Sutherland et al., "Adaptation to the Dry Colostomy: Preliminary Report and Summary of Findings," *The Psychological Impact of Cancer* (American Cancer Society Professional Education Publication), pp. 1-16. See p. 5.

24. A.M. Sutherland and C.E. Orbach, "Depressive Reactions Associated with Surgery for Cancer," *The Psychological Impact of Cancer* (op. cit.), pp. 17-21. See pp. 17-18.

25. Ibid., pp. 17-19.

26. Ibid., p. 18.

27. Sutherland et al., op. cit., p. 13.

28. Ibid.

29. Ibid., p. 14.

30. McIntosh, op. cit., p. 169.

31. Oken, op. cit., pp. 1124-1125.

32. Ibid., p. 1125

33. F. Davis, op. cit. See p. 319.

34. D. Sudnow, *Passing on: The Social Organization of Dying* (Englewood Cliffs, N.J.: Prentice-Hall, 1967). See pp. 68-69 for discussion of this issue.

35. E.C. Easson, "Cancer and the Problem of Pessimism," *Cancer* 17 (1967): 7-14.

36. B.G. Glaser and A.L. Strauss, *Awareness of Dying* (Chicago: Aldine Publishing Co., 1965).

37. McIntosh, op. cit., pp. 178-179.

38. J.C. Quint, "Mastectomy—Symbol of Cure or Warning Sign?" *General Practice* 29 (1964): 119.

※ *Chapter 7*

# Prospects and Problems in Cancer Screening

One of the great truisms with which Americans have approached cancer over the last quarter century is that early detection and treatment are the most effective measures that can be taken against the disease. Few would dispute the value of early detection, and many individuals today periodically undergo screening procedures designed to detect the presence of malignancies before they have developed far enough to produce visible symptoms. The National Cancer Act expressly mandates public support for cancer detection and encourages the establishment of public screening facilities for this purpose.[1] But, as the preceding chapters have argued in other aspects of cancer control such as diffusing new knowledge among physicians, upgrading the functions of nurses, and providing patients with emotional support, only limited progress appears possible within the pattern of social relations presently governing health care. Like most health care facilities in the cancer control program service region, those that specialize in cancer detection are organized independently of other health care providers. Independent organization and specialized function, two important features of the social technology utilized by health care providers today, limit the contribution that early detection can make to cancer control.

The discussion to follow does not dispute the technical potential of cancer screening. The ten-year survival rate for some of the most common cancers—buccal, larynx, colon, breast, uterine, ovarian, kidney, bladder, and lymph node malignancies—is 30 percent higher among patients in whom the disease is diagnosed while still localized than among those in whom it is widely diffused.[2] Insead, the present chapter argues that neither the construction of new screening facilities, nor the augmentation of public access to existing ones, nor even improved detection procedures in doctors' offices can increase the proportion of cancers detected while still localized to its technically feasible maximum. Despite the enthusiastic support by public and private health authorities for early detection, many facilities established for this purpose have failed. Reflecting on this discouraging observation, one specialist in early cancer detection commented:

> We should have been learning what it takes to get people into early detection facilities and what it takes to get people to comply with preventive medicine recommendations. While we were building computer programs we should have also been developing outreach mechanisms to get high risk patients into early detection facilities. Instead of 12, 14, or 16 channel autoanalyzers, we should have been developing a meaningful followup system with end result evaluation.[3]

This observer's comments summarize the difficulties that prevent health professionals and the public from realizing the full benefits possible under existing cancer detection technology. As the quotation suggests, mere availability of cancer detection facilities does not insure utilization. Many individuals who could benefit from early detection appear unlikely to make use of facilities established for this purpose. The members of the population least strongly inclined to seek early detection, moreover, may be those with the most to gain from such procedures. As Chapter 3 notes, cancer incidence and mortality are highest among poor people and racial minorities both in the Central City University Cancer Control Program service region and the United States as a whole. But an extensive series of investigations strongly suggests that the most consistent users of preventive health care facilities like cancer screening tend to be educated, socially advantaged, and white. In a survey of preventive health behavior, for example, Colburn and Pope report that individuals with the highest incomes and levels of education were most likely to receive vaccination for polio and to visit physicians and dentists for precautionary and preventive purposes.[4] The findings of this investigation imply that income (and hence availability of medical services) explains only part of the individual's inclination to seek preventive health care. While individuals with the highest incomes showed the strongest tendency to seek physical examinations, those with the highest levels of education sought polio vaccinations most often. Several investigations focusing specifically on cancer reveal highly similar phenomena. Kutner and Gordon, for example, report that individuals with low levels of education, income, and socioeconomic status exhibit a tendency to delay seeking care in response to symptoms of illness. Kutner and Gordon's data indicate that the tendency of socially disadvantaged people to delay seeking medical care is even stronger among those who experience one of cancer's "seven warning signals."[5] And in an important study of the HIP breast cancer screening program in New York City, Fink reports that those who participated tended to be younger and better educated than those who stayed away.[6] Although early detection may currently be gaining wider public acceptability, the population segments among which it is most widely accepted may face the lowest levels of risk. Evidence suggesting that only restricted categories of people like the well educated and economically secure utilized cancer screening facilities would present planners with serious problems.

A second question integrally related to the benefits society may or may not draw from large-scale early detection programs concerns the speed and efficiency with which members of the public and health professionals respond to indications of malignancies generated through early detection procedures. Early detection of cancer symptoms typically takes place in locations and settings different from definitive diagnosis and treatment. Even the select group of individuals who do seek early detection of cancer through periodic examinations in a doctor's office or multiphasic screening procedures will draw scant benefits from this activity if they are unwilling or unable to move promptly toward definitive diagnosis and therapy. As is typically the case with modern disease, the ability of the individual with cancer to benefit from medical treatment often appears to depend strongly on the ability to move swiftly and efficiently from point to point within the health care system.

The activity or inactivity of physicians may play an important part in whether early detection procedures actually benefit people who partake of them. Several researchers on cancer detection and treatment have identified physician-related factors that contribute to delay in the process by which patients reach sources of definitive care. Makover, for example, identifies the concept of "physician delay" as the prolonging of diagnosis and therapy beyond what can be reasonably expected from current standards of medical practice.[7] A classical study of delay in reaching definitive treatment among cancer patients reported that 17 percent of the patients studied were delayed by their doctors and another 18 percent, while contributing to delay themselves, were subject to physician-initiated delay as well. Physician delay was defined here as failure either to reach a diagnosis or to make proper referral within one month of the patient's first visit.[8] Makover suggests that "organizational factors" including method of payment, lack of convenient laboratory facilities, and the need to refer patients to distantly located consultants contribute to the reluctance of some physicians to begin definitive treatment or refer patients elsewhere.[9]

Research not specifically related to cancer suggests additional factors that may inhibit patients from reaching the source of care that may benefit them most. Physicians may catagorically reject findings based on standardized testing procedures such as those that characterize multiphasic health screening.[10] Furthermore, referral relationships among physicians may make it difficult for patients to reach appropriate diagnosticians and therapists. As Shortell and Anderson document in general medicine[11] and Chapter 4 of this volume shows in the context of cancer-related services, status differences, breaches of professional courtesy, and fear of income loss may inhibit or short-circuit referral.

Most research on delay in definitive diagnosis and treatment for illness of all kinds focuses not on the organization of health care, but on the patient. Several investigators report, for example, that a variety of personal characteristics inhibit individuals from making initial contacts with health care providers. In his well-known conceptualization of the sick role, Parsons writes that "most normal people . . . are motivated to underestimate their chances of falling ill, especially seriously ill."[12] Empirical researchers have reported many attitudinal and social structural variables that discourage individuals from viewing themselves as ill and seeking professional help. Koos writes that given similar symptoms, lower class persons are less inclined than upper class persons to think that they are ill and to consult physicians.[13] Suchman implies that many consider themselves ill and in need of help only if they experience obvious need in the form of pain and other "severe, continuous, incapacitating, and unalleviated" symptoms.[14] Mechanic lists psychological factors including stigmatization, social distance, and feelings of humiliation along with such concrete items as time, money, and effort as deterrents to seeking help in health care.[15] Emphasizing concrete variables, Andersen notes that individuals are often unlikely to seek medical care in the absence of "enabling factors" such as personal, family, and community resources.[16] Aday adds that those who have no regular source of medical care are less likely to see physicians in response to disabling illness than those who do.[17]

Even after initial contact with physicians, similar factors often motivate patients not to comply with medical regimens. In a review of an extensive literature, Becker and Maiman suggest that patients who do not perceive their symptoms as serious are less likely to follow physicians' instructions than those convinced that they are or may become seriously ill.[18] Battistella notes that individuals who are optimistic about the ability of medicine to successfully treat serious illness are less likely to delay recommended treatment than others.[19] Korsch states that weak doctor-patient relationships, appearing as poor communication or unfulfilled expectations, increase both delay and noncompliance.[20]

The factors associated with delay in the patient's approach to health care providers and noncompliance with medical regimens seem likely to occur in cancer detection as well, especially when early detection activities take the form of automated, multiphasic health screening procedures. Several features of automated, multiphasic examinations appear likely to attenuate doctor-patient relationships and discourage prompt patient follow-up. Davis reports that administration of large numbers of tests in general medicine tends to discourage compliance with medical directives.[21] According to several studies, health professionals who have no regular association with their patients—a characteristic of doctors at screening centers—command less authority over their acts than family physicians.[22] Cancer, though, is sufficiently different from other diseases to caution the investigator against automatically assuming the applicability of findings observed in other illnesses. The dread with which most people perceive cancer seems likely to cause many to delay seeking conclusive diagnosis when informed of suspicious indications, a factor that encourages victims of other illnesses to seek help.[23]

The literature on health care services, particularly preventive health behavior, suggests that planners and social scientists are likely to encounter serious problems in establishing large-scale facilities for the early detection of cancer. To assist the scholar and planner in understanding the behavioral factors that might prevent a regional system of installations established specifically for the early detection of cancer on a mass basis from materially affecting the cancer morbidity and mortality rates, this chapter provides a detailed examination of an important feature of patient behavior in a large, well-established cancer detection facility: patient-initiated delay in obtaining definitive diagnosis and treatment following notification of positive findings in screening procedures. The problem of patient-initiated delay is, of course, only one of the three difficulties that the health care literature suggests will hamper the efficiency of large-scale cancer screening. The emphasis given this difficulty in the present chapter does not imply that physician-initiated delay or differential self-selection of the population for early cancer detection are problems of lesser importance. In keeping with the major perspective of this volume, however, an examination of the actions of individuals already making use of a cancer detection facility is particularly useful. This chapter will point out connections between seemingly independent decisions and actions taken by individuals following their visits to a cancer screening center and (1) the methods employed by organizations performing cancer-related services and (2) the relationship of the specialized screening facility to the health care system as a whole.

## THE METROPOLITAN SCREENING CLINIC

The Metropolitan Screening Clinic, a large, well-established early detection facility for cancer in Central City, provided an unusual opportunity for researchers to study the attitudes and behavior of people faced with the possibility of having cancer and the necessity of seeking definitive diagnosis and treatment. Faced with extremely frightening possibilities, the individuals who attend the clinic in search of early detection of malignancies and receive word of positive findings would appear quite likely to seek ways of avoiding taking the necessary action. As a health care facility, the clinic is highly unusual because, although it defines its function as detecting the possibility of malignancies, it specifically excludes definitive diagnosis of cancer or therapy for malignant conditions from its repertoire of services. The individual who undergoes screening—referred to by clinic personnel as a "screenee" rather than a patient—has the responsibility of independently procuring definitive diagnosis and treatment from physicians outside the facility. While an unusual health care organization, the clinic typifies the automated, multiphasic operation that many planners see as the most efficient method of reducing the mortality rate from cancer by detecting the disease in its early stages through publicly financed mass screening.

The Metropolitan Screening Clinic (a fictitious name for an actual facility) was founded in the 1930s. It is perhaps the oldest facility established specifically for the detection of cancer, and it ranks among the first organizations to perform automated screening procedures for diseases of any kind. Located on Central City's west side, the clinic is only a short walk from the most fashionable part of the central business district and choice residential areas on the river front. Because of the near juxtaposition of wealth and poverty that characterizes many parts of Central City, though, the clinic faces a zone of somewhat dilapidated housing and business establishments across a busy arterial street. Occupying a low-rise building of poured concrete, the facilities strike visitors as austere and drab, particularly in winter. While the clinic is outside the official boundaries of the cancer control program service region, the distance from it is not great. Individuals who live on the city's east side or in Home County enjoy reliable public transportation to the central business district and are often willing to make the sacrifices necessary to utilize the clinic's services.

The clinic's examining procedure parallels that of many other automated, multiphasic health screening activities in existence today, such as, for example, that of the Kaiser system in California. Screenees at Metropolitan undergo an extensive battery of tests, including most standardized cancer detection procedures such as X-rays, proctoscopy, and mammography. The battery requires less than three hours to complete and in 1977, cost the screenee $80.00. The clinic screens about 2,000 people every month, uncovers suspicious symptoms among about 12 percent of them, and, in an average year, discovers approximately 120 proven cases of cancer. Screenees generally report a high level of satisfaction with the procedure, and many come back for retesting at regular intervals of from one to three years. Although Metropolitan aims primarily at detecting cancers at asymptomatic stages, screenees are informed when they show signs of other illnesses or abnormalities. The clinic's program includes such noncancer-related procedures as hearing and vision testing, an electrocardiogram, and a test for diabetes. The screening begins with a set of health history questions that, like most of the clinic's functions, is mechanized. Screenees respond to questions appearing on a television screen by pressing buttons on a typewriterlike computer input device. Physicians perform complete physical examinations on all clients and conduct certain specialized procedures, while nurses and technicians administer many of the other tests.

Although the clinic's examination procedure should seem familiar to those who have undergone multiphasic screening elsewhere, the methods by which screenees receive information about the results of the examination may differ. At any time during the screening, a physician may inform the screenee of a suspicious finding. Screenees have the option of returning to the clinic for a consultation with the physician when its personnel have completed analysis of the test results. Physicians tend to inform patients of possible problems at the examination only for obvious findings, otherwise reserving their comments for consultation sessions. Screenees who do not attend the consultations receive a letter from the clinic informing them, if appropriate, of suspicious findings in general language. If the screenee has listed the name of a regular family physician on the intake form, the clinic sends the physician a copy of its test results in the form of a computer printout. The clinic attempts to keep track of the responses of its screenees to findings indicating the possibility of cancer, sending forms to their physicians asking whether they have examined the screenee. When screenees with suspicious findings name no regular physician, they receive requests to inform the clinic of the name of the physician they do see. The clinic considers a suspicious case "closed" only when it receives confirmation from a physician that the screenee has been examined. The clinic mails up to four reminders to both screenee and physician if no physician return form is returned.

A serious concern with the possibility that many screenees were not, in fact, consulting physicians in response to positive findings from the clinic led its directors to invite academic researchers into their organization. According to Metropolitan's records, 35 percent of the cases in which the clinic had detected indications of possible cancers remained unclosed. If this rate of incomplete follow-up meant that an equivalent percentage of screenees with suspicious findings ignored communications from the clinic or never consulted physicians, Metropolitan would face serious problems indeed. Even the most perfectly developed technical means of detecting cancer would save no lives under its system of patient-initiated follow-up if the screenees took no action in response to the clinic findings.

Of course, the percentage of cases remaining unclosed in Metropolitan's records might have indicated no cause for genuine alarm. Informed of suspicious findings, these screenees might take immediate action, locating the best possible care for their suspected malignancy. The physician selected for this purpose may well have been a practitioner different from the one named, and the patient, understandably preoccupied with his or her physical condition, may have forgotten to request that the physician inform the Metropolitan Screening Clinic of his or her visit. Alternatively, the physician's office, already burdened with large volumes of paperwork from public agencies, insurance companies, and the like, may place low priority on returning the forms it receives from Metropolitan. While the clinic occasionally contacts screenees by telephone, it ordinarily follows up cases by sending letters at periodic intervals to screenees and doctors, closing cases only when the doctors reply. While understandable, the patient's or physician's neglect of Metropolitan's reporting procedure may leave the names of numerous screenees who have taken prompt and appropriate action among the clinic's backlog of unclosed cases.

The present study attempted to determine what percentage of Metropolitan's unclosed cases actually represented individuals who failed to seek definitive care in response to its findings, to learn why those who failed to comply with the clinic directives avoided action, and to identify other problems in the clinic's functioning by studying a sample of unclosed cases in its files. The clinic made available 430 unclosed case records; we attempted to contact all these individuals by telephone, eventually reached 300 of them, and performed short interviews over the telephone covering demographic characteristics, attitudes about Metropolitan, and activity in response to its findings. Researchers attempted to perform face-to-face interviews with as many of those who reported never having seen a doctor in response to Metropolitan's findings as resources permitted. Interviewers eventually completed thirty of these personal interviews, which usually lasted between one and two hours. Both the telephone and direct interviewing employed standardized research tools, specimens of which appear along with the Professional Community Survey in the appendix.

According to the telephone survey, the worst suspicions of Metropolitan's directors did not seem to be borne out. The survey included items that asked, first, whether the respondent had procured medical care, and if so, how much time elapsed between receiving the letter from Metropolitan and visiting the physician. Of the 300 individuals who answered, only 16 percent had not seen doctors in response to letters and consultations at Metropolitan. Many screenees who contacted their physicians, though, did so only after extended periods of delay. As Table 7-1 shows, only about 40 percent of the sample contacted a doctor within two weeks of receiving the first letter from Metropolitan. We adopted a working definition of noncompliance

**Table 7-1. Time Elapsed Between Notification of Symptoms and Medical Follow-up**

| Time Elapsed Before Follow-up | Percentage of Sample |
|---|---|
| 0–2 weeks | 40.8 (118) |
| 3–11 weeks | 29.8 (87) |
| 12–15 weeks | 5.8 (17) |
| 16 weeks or longer (includes indefinite) | 24.0 (70) |
| | 100% = (292) |

that included all screenees who delayed sixteen weeks or longer as well as those who never contacted physicians. According to these criteria, 24 percent, or seventy individuals, were noncompliers. On the basis of this finding, we estimated a total noncompliance rate of 8.4 percent among all individuals in whom Metropolitan detected indications of cancer. The 300 persons reached in the telephone survey were drawn from a pool representing 35 percent of the clinic's suspicious cases. The total percentage of noncompliers appeared to be 24 percent of this pool, or 8.4 percent of the total of individuals with positive findings.

The telephone survey, however, did provide indications that the clinic faced several important barriers to successful completion of its mission. The most obvious problem that these data suggest is that the clinic's method of tracking its clientele is faulty. Apparently, many screenees and doctors do neglect or ignore the reporting procedure. This difficulty not only generates an overestimate of nonfollow-up among the clinic's caseload, but also may discourage its decisionmakers from formulating a special outreach effort designed to reach those who do not comply with its directives. Assuming the task to be too great for their resources, they may decide to formulate no outreach procedure at all.

By providing a glimpse at the segment of the Central City regional population most likely to utilize the clinic services, the telephone survey suggests a second problem in the organization's functioning. As the literature on preventive health care suggests, only a restricted part of the population seems to utilize the clinic services. According to Table 7-2, education plays a strong part in the decision to seek cancer screening at Metropolitan. Individuals with eight years or fewer of education constituted almost 27 percent of the population of the Central City SMSA according to the 1970 census. Only 7 percent of the persons interviewed in the telephone survey, however, reported that they had attended school for eight years or less. On the other end of the scale, fewer than 12 percent of the residents of the Central City SMSA reported that they had attended four or more years of college to the 1970 census. But over 30 percent of those responding to the telephone survey indicated that they had received four or more years of college education. At least within the population sampled in the telephone interviews, college graduates are overrepresented by nearly 300 percent in comparison with the population of the surrounding region.

If these statistics reflected the educational composition of the clinic users as a whole, they would indicate that the services it offered were attractive to only the more educated segments of the

Table 7-2.  Level of Education Among Metropolitan Clinic Screenees and Residents of Central City SMSA[a]

| Educational Level | Metropolitan Screenees | Central City SMSA[b] |
|---|---|---|
| 8 years and under | 6.8 | 26.6 |
| High School: | | |
| 1–3 years | 9.7 | 19.5 |
| 4 years | 27.0 | 30.7 |
| College | | |
| 1–3 years | 25.2 | 11.5 |
| 4 years or more | 31.3 | 11.7 |
| 100% = | (278) | (6,978,967) |

[a]Entries in table are percentages in groups with various levels of education.
[b]Source of Central City SMSA data: U.S. Census, Census of Population and Housing: 1970 U.S. Table includes data on Central City residents 25 years of age and over.

region's population. Although the telephone survey sampled only clinic screenees who (1) received word that they might have cancer and (2) never, according to the clinic records, visited a physician, this generalization is tempting to make. Many individuals who did, in fact, obtain medical care in response to the clinic directives remained in the file of unclosed cases. Apparently, the presence of a name in this file may have resulted from faults in the clinic's reporting system as easily as the screenee's personal, social, or disease characteristics. The fact that a screenee's name remained in the file of unclosed cases, for example, could have as much to do with the selection of a physician without sufficient clerical assistance to return the form as with the patient's reluctance to comply with the clinic recommendations. The selection procedure that yielded names for the telephone survey, then, implies that the overrepresentation of individuals who delayed or avoided seeing a physician was small or nonexistent. The characteristics of the clinic reporting system, then, form the basis of a strong case that the telephone sample represents not those who received word of suspicious symptoms and took no action, but *all* screenees in whom the clinic detected indications of possible cancer. Unless we are willing to assume that advanced education is strongly connected with cancer symptoms, we may infer that the educated residents of the Central City region are far more likely to utilize the clinic services than their less educated neighbors.

According to this argument, though, racial minorities are not underrepresented in the clinic's population. While nonwhites consti-

Table 7-3. Racial Composition of Metropolitan Clinic Screenees and Residents of Central City SMSA[a]

| Race | Metropolitan Center | Central City SMSA[b] |
|------|---------------------|----------------------|
| White | 75.6 | 81.2 |
| Black | 21.0 | 17.6 |
| Other | 3.4 | 1.2 |
| 100% = | (289) | (6,978,947) |

[a]Entries in table are percentages of racial groupings among Metropolitan Center screenees and residents of Central City.
[b]Source: See Table 7-2.

tute 18.8 percent of the region's population, they composed 24 percent of the respondents to the telephone survey (see Table 7-3). A strong tendency of racial minorities to delay or avoid medical consultations would explain their overrepresentation in this sample. But, as discussion to follow will indicate, our research shows no significant relation between racial characteristics and delay. One possibility consistent with the data in Table 7-3 is that nonwhites utilize the clinic more frequently in response to visible symptoms than whites. This possibility, which will receive detailed attention in the discussion to follow, indicates a second problem that the clinic may face in achieving its goal of detecting cancers before they become visible to individuals as symptoms; that is, some categories of clinic users may seek the organization's services only *after* the appearance of visible signs associated with cancer.

The characteristics of the telephone survey sample, of course, add a strong element of speculation to these observations. They add weight to the suspicion generated by previous research in preventive health behavior that the socially disadvantaged would be relatively unlikely to utilize cancer screening facilities even though they have more to gain from these resources than the socially advantaged. We are on far safer ground, however, in commenting on the problem that originally led the clinic directors to intiate the research. Assuming that the telephone survey sample accurately represents the clinic's backlog of unclosed cases, 8.4 percent of the screenees who receive word that they may have cancer are *noncompliers*, that is, individuals who engage in lengthy delays before seeing physicians or who avoid medical attention entirely. Although the clinic initially overestimated this percentage, they still detected a serious problem.

Even a "small" percentage of individuals in whom detection facilities identified indications of cancer and who did not seek prompt medical attention implies that many deaths from cancer may occur needlessly. This problem may constitute the most serious ultimate barrier to successful mass screening efforts. The present study, then, concentrated on determining why individuals often do delay or avoid taking action in response to the clinic directives.

The telephone survey sample is well suited for an investigation of this problem. As suggested above, the sample constitutes a set of compliers and noncompliers selected in a highly similar manner. Without assuming that this sample represents the clinic's total clientele or any other concrete universe of individuals, it provides a basis for the identification of at least some of the individual attributes, social attributes, and disease characteristics associated with noncompliance.

## FACTORS AFFECTING COMPLIANCE AND DELAY

Both the telephone survey and personal interviews provided data useful in explaining why many patients fail to seek medical consultations in response to Metropolitan's directives and why others delay taking action. The telephone and face-to-face interview schedules approach this problem from differing perspectives. The telephone interviews were intended to be large in number and specific in focus. Based on a few questions calling for specific answers, the telephone interviewing aimed at providing data that are easily quantifiable and transferable directly from forms used by interviewers to forms that can be read by the computer. Data of this nature are most suitable for testing specific hypotheses suggested in the health services literature about the noncompliance problem in cancer screening. Barring the introduction of elaborate mathematical representations of the data, however, a highly focused investigation of this kind can only produce a broad outline of the phenomenon. The discovery of statistically significant relationships among numerical variables, furthermore, gives the reader no firm indication of the processes that these relationships reflect. The face-to-face interviewing is designed to fill the gaps left by the statistical analysis. This part of the investigation included relatively few observations and questions that were purposely broad in scope. Items on the personal interviewing instrument were intended to parallel the "depth" format most familiar in therapeutic settings. Questions of this type encourage respondents to tell of personal feelings and recall specific experiences that are difficult to capture through highly focused questioning procedures. Although the face-to-face procedure used here did not generate numerical data or provide the basis for determining statistically significant relationships, it suggested concrete interpretations of the statistical relationships determined with the aid of the telephone procedure.

The nature of both cancer and the process of health screening necessitates this two-pronged research approach. Health screening is a more complex phenomenon than visiting a physician or otherwise initiating health care. It is a preliminary step that must be followed up to be effective. The search for simple correlations between attitude, personality, and social position, on the one hand, and preventive health behavior, on the other, is inadequate because of the complexity of the process. The screenee's reaction to positive findings from early detection procedures is, of course, the pivotal phenomenon to be investigated. But attributes of the screenee that preceded the screening process are likely to influence these reactions. The complexity of cancer diagnosis and treatment as social processes renders analyses of these activities complex themselves. While studies of noncompliance in treatment of acute conditions have focused on the patient's relationship with a single physician, the linkage between screening and diagnosis implies that the screenee's relations with at least two sets of health professionals are crucial in determining follow-up behavior. Attitudes and capacities that lead individuals to initiate the screening process cannot be assumed to speed the initiation of medical follow-up to positive findings. While the Metropolitan Screening Clinic is a highly visible, well-advertised facility in the Central City region, for example, definitive cancer-related medical services may be considerably more difficult to locate. Finding a screening center, then, is a markedly different task from finding a physician specially skilled in cancer diagnosis or treatment. Events at the screening procedure may change attitudes about preventive health care related to cancer. In general, the multiplicity of interrelated factors that appear likely to affect speed of follow-up requires the researcher to adopt a multifaceted approach to the investigation.

Although the final analysis of delay and noncompliance in cancer screening must include much data of the "soft" variety, including especially striking testimony by individual screenees, the investigation here begins with a statistical analysis. This analysis serves as the basis for all conclusions that will eventually be presented. Because the questions posed here are more complex than in preceding chapters, the accompanying statistical analysis is more complex as well.

The qualitatively inclined reader may wish to concentrate mainly on less standardized data presented later in the chapter. While the statistical analysis adds reliability and rigor to the conclusions, readers may gain an adequate understanding of problems related to cancer screening on the basis of the extensive interviewing that accompanied the systematic survey.

### Statistical Explanations of Delay

The statistical investigation of delay and noncompliance is based on closed-ended questions in the telephone survey. The interview schedule used in this part of the study of the Metropolitan Screening Clinic included items designed to measure factors associated in the health care literature with behavior similar to medical follow-up in cancer screening. The questionnaire administered during the telephone interview generated numerical indications of each respondent's attitudes toward health care, relationships with the health care system, and social background characteristics. We expected that these factors would at least partially explain the amount of time each screenee required to obtain medical follow-up, a variable also measured by an item on the telephone interview schedule.

It is immediately evident that at least some of these factors explained the screenee's tendency to delay or avoid visiting a physician in response to Metropolitan's directive. According to Table 7-4, for instance, screenees who listed a family physician on their intake forms at the clinic delayed contacting a physician significantly less than those who listed none. Respondents who reported relatively recent visits to a physician also tended to delay follow-up less than others. The small number of respondents ($N = 12$) who were referred to the clinic by health care providers tended to avoid delay, as did those who cited a "periodic routine to maintain good health" as an important reason for seeking screening, those with several relatives who had had cancer, and those with relatively high occupational status measured according to a slightly modified version of Blau and Duncan's classification scheme.[24] The table shows little if any relation between delay and attending the clinic in response to symptoms of illness, satisfaction with the clinic, recommendation by the clinic for surgical consultation, age, race, level of education, and marital status.

Table 7-4 appears to indicate that three variables related to contact with the health care system (listing a regular physician, having recently visited a physician, and having been referred by a provider), one attitudinal variable (considering periodic, routine checkups an important reason for attending Metropolitan), and one social back-

Table 7-4.   Coefficients of Correlation (Pearson) Among Variables Related to Delay in Follow-up[a]

|  | (1) | (2) | (3) | (4) | (5) | (6) | (7) | (8) | (9) | (10) | (11) | (12) | (13) | (14) |
|---|---|---|---|---|---|---|---|---|---|---|---|---|---|---|
| (1) Delay | — | | | | | | | | | | | | | |
| (2) Lists regular physician | -.32 | — | | | | | | | | | | | | |
| (3) Recent visit to physician | -.16 | .18 | — | | | | | | | | | | | |
| (4) Periodic checkups important | -.11 | .11 | .22 | — | | | | | | | | | | |
| (5) Had symptoms | .03 | .03 | .06 | -.19 | — | | | | | | | | | |
| (6) Referred by provider | -.16 | .07 | -.01 | -.16 | .22 | — | | | | | | | | |
| (7) Number of cancers in family | -.11 | .07 | .04 | .01 | -.01 | -.01 | — | | | | | | | |
| (8) Satisfaction with clinic | -.02 | -.04 | .01 | -.02 | -.07 | .00 | -.04 | — | | | | | | |
| (9) Surgical consult recommended | -.04 | .08 | .10 | .07 | .01 | -.07 | .04 | -.03 | — | | | | | |
| (10) Occupation | -.17 | .08 | -.01 | .11 | -.05 | -.10 | .17 | .06 | -.06 | — | | | | |
| (11) Age | -.06 | .21 | -.05 | -.02 | -.03 | .06 | -.04 | .01 | .10 | .01 | — | | | |
| (12) White | -.04 | .10 | -.14 | -.14 | -.10 | -.03 | .16 | -.10 | -.07 | .00 | .13 | — | | |
| (13) Level of education | -.02 | -.04 | -.05 | .08 | -.09 | -.09 | .06 | -.10 | -.01 | .52 | -.30 | -.01 | — | |
| (14) Married | -.03 | .05 | .01 | .03 | -.03 | -.02 | .06 | .18 | -.04 | .03 | .09 | .01 | -.03 | — |

[a]$p < .05$ for all coefficients of .10 or greater.

ground variable (occupational status) are the major determinants of prompt follow-up. To test the robustness of these relations, all five variables were entered in a series of regression equations (see Table 7-5). The first equation (equation *A*) also includes age and educational level, background variables that explain much behavior and thought, and the number of cancer cases that had occurred among the respondent's blood relations. None of these variables was significant in equation *A*, and when dropped to produce equation *B* decreased the amount of variance explained only slightly. Under the assumption that all important relations in this system are linear, equation *C* in Table 7-5 constitutes the most efficient model to explain delay in follow-up. In this equation, the three items related to contact with the health care system and the single background variable of occupational status explain nearly as much variance in delay as the less parsimonious equation *A*.

Although it is undeniable that contact with the health care system and occupational status explain a major portion of the variance in delay, the conclusion that attitudinal and experiential factors are unimportant is premature. Like most survey data, analysis of responses to the telephone interviews reveals interactive and nonlinear relations. As Table 7-6 shows, a meaningful relation between considering periodic, routine checkups an important reason for attending the clinic and prompt follow-up exists only among individuals who report that two or more cancers have occurred among their

**Table 7-5. Standardized Partial Regression Coefficients from Equations Predicting Delay in Medical Follow-up: Linear Relations Only**

| | Beta Weights | | |
|---|---|---|---|
| *Independent Variables* | *(A)* | *(B)* | *(C)* |
| Lists regular physician | $-.27^a$ | $-.27^a$ | $-.28^a$ |
| Recent visit to physician | $-.10$ | $-.10$ | $-.12^b$ |
| Periodic checkups important | $-.07$ | $-.06$ | — |
| Referred by provider | $-.16^a$ | $-.16^b$ | $-.15^a$ |
| Occupation | $-.18^a$ | $-.15^a$ | $-.16^a$ |
| Age | $.01$ | — | |
| Level of education | $.06$ | — | |
| Number of cancers in family | $-.06$ | — | |
| | $R^2 = .17$ | $R^2 = .16$ | $R^2 = .16$ |

[a] $p < .01.$
[b] $p < .05.$

Table 7-6. Percentage Delaying Follow-up Two Weeks or Less by Importance of Periodic, Routine Checkups, Controlling for Number of Cancers Among Blood Relations

| | Consider Periodic, Routine Checkups Important | |
|---|---|---|
| *Number of Cancers in Family* | *Yes* | *No* |
| 0-1 | 40.6 (63) | 37.9 (25) |
| 2 or more[a] | 57.6 (19) | 25.0  (4) |

[a]$p < .10.$

Table 7-7. Relation Between Importance of Periodic, Routine Checkups and Delay in Follow-up

| | | Importance of Periodic, Routine Checkups | | |
|---|---|---|---|---|
| | | *Low* | *Medium* | *High* |
| | 0-2 weeks | 36.2 | 22.6 | 46.6 |
| Delay in Contacting Physician | 3-11 weeks | 32.5 | 29.0 | 27.3 |
| | Over 12 weeks or never | 31.3 | 48.4 | 26.1 |
| | 100% = | (80) | (31) | (161) |

Gamma = -0.17, $p < .10.$

blood relations. Table 7-7 demonstrates that attributing importance to the periodic routine is related to delay in a curvilinear manner, those who consider routine examination of moderate importance tending to delay follow-up longer than either those who consider the routine very important or slightly important.

The equations in Table 7-8 demonstrate the statistical significance of these nonlinear relations even when all other variables have explained all they can. Equation A in Table 7-8 contains an "interaction term" whose magnitude is the value the respondent places on periodic examinations when one or more cancers have occurred in the family and zero when none has occurred. The interaction term is significant at the .05 level, even when the three most important predictors of delay that appeared in Table 7-5 (listing a regular physician, attending Metropolitan at the suggestion of a provider, and occupational status) are included in the same equation.

Similarly, a term representing the curvilinear relation between

Table 7-8. Standardized Partial Regression Coefficients from Equations Predicting Delay in Medical Follow-up: Models Including Interactions and Nonlinear Relations

| Independent Variables | Beta Weights | |
| --- | --- | --- |
|  | (A) | (B) |
| Lists regular physician | $-.30^a$ | $-.28^a$ |
| Referred by provider | $-.16^a$ | $-.14^a$ |
| Occupation | $-.14^b$ | $-.15^a$ |
| Recent visit to physician | — | $-.12^b$ |
| Periodic checkups important (quadratic representation) | — | $-.12^b$ |
| Periodic checkups important (interaction with number of cancers in family) | $-.13^b$ | — |
|  | $R^2 = .16$ | $R = .18$ |

$^a p < .01.$
$^b p < .05.$

valuation of periodic examinations and delay is statistically significant even after several other variables have explained all they can. Equation *B* in Table 7-8 represents the value individuals place upon periodic examinations as the outcome variable of a quadratic equation of the following form:

$$y = 1 + 3x + x^2$$

where $x$ equals the value respondents place on periodic examinations according to the four-point scale used in the questionnaire format. The quadratic equation creates a new variable representing valuation of examinations, in which the inverted U-shaped relation depicted in Table 7-7 between delay and valuation of examinations is transformed into a straight line. This procedure, which allows a nonlinear relation to be examined by computer algorithms restricted to linear relations, demonstrates that the individual's valuation of periodic examinations is significant at the .05 level in predicting delay.

It seems reasonable to conclude from Table 7-8 that some attitudinal and experiential variables do help explain delay of medical follow-up among the Metropolitan clinic screenees. The tendency of those who report cancer deaths among their blood relations and at the same time value periodic checkups not to delay suggests that perceived threat promotes prompt contact. The importance of belief in periodic checkups is more complex, individuals with middle-level commitments delaying significantly more than those with weak or strong commitments. The equations in Table 7-8, though, still indicate that regular contact with the health care system, or specifically with doctors, is most important in determining length of delay. It is noteworthy that the twelve individuals who reported that health care providers referred them to the clinic all indicated that these providers were doctors, usually their regular family physicians. Face-to-face interviewing provided amplification of the role the screenee's contact with physicians plays in determining delay.

### Personal Experiences and Explanations

Face-to-face interviews of Metropolitan screenees who never followed up their visits or did so after a sixteen-week delay yielded much valuable data on noncompliance. These data, of course, are much less standardized than those presented in the statistical analysis. If considered in isolation, many analysts would argue that this interview material was essentially speculative, capable of generating hypotheses for further research but not of supporting conclusions. The face-to-face interviews of noncompliers in this research, though, are necessary to make the statistical data meaningful. The feelings and experiences that the subjects described specify the range of meanings captured by formal questionnaire items. Information of this kind, furthermore, provides evidence of relationships too complex to be conveniently expressed by multiple regression models. Finally, the interview data do generate hypotheses valuable not only to future researchers, but also worthy of consideration by planners in decisionmaking where incomplete information prevails.

The face-to-face interviews, for example, demonstrate several specific meanings that may be connected with the statistical association between relations with the health care system and compliance. The statistical model in Table 7-8, once again, indicates that those who have regular physicians, receive referrals from health professionals (i.e., physicians) to the clinic, or report recent visits to physicians are the most likely to seek prompt medical follow-up in response to positive findings. The responses of persons interviewed personally suggest more specific features of the patient's relation with the health care system that lead to noncompliance and delay.

One theme that emerged in the interviewing strongly suggested that lack of access to physicians contributed to delay or avoidance of medical follow-up in response to the clinic findings. Respondents in the face-to-face interviews suggested several problems, ranging from simply being unable to obtain physicians' services to feeling dissatisfied with the quality of care that was available to them. Several non-compliers told us that they had not been able to locate "good family doctors" following the retirement or death of their regular primary care physicians or relocation to their current locale. Some interview subjects explained their noncompliance as inability to find a regular source of medical care. One recent migrant to the region decried the fact that he had not located a "reliable" physician since his arrival and wished that Metropolitan maintained a "list of good doctors" for screenees to contact when their examination indicated the necessity. Two ghetto dwellers reported similar, concrete difficulties in following up Metropolitan's recommendations. One indicated that she had not followed up because the only primary care facility in her neighborhood was a "Medicaid Mill," which she preferred to avoid. The other indicated that a primary care clinic existed in her neighborhood, connected with a local hospital. She was reluctant to attend this clinic, though, because it did not provide care by the same physician on successive visits. Finally, one woman told us she had made a conscientious yet frustrating attempt to procure a surgical consultation after Metropolitan informed her of a suspicious mammogram. The respondent said she had gone to a large clinic for the consultation but had encountered so many "bureaucratic procedures," seeing "everybody but a doctor," that she abandoned the effort.

Noncompliers raised another theme in the face-to-face interviews that seemed consistent with the multiple regression analysis. Several mentioned that although simple access to physicians had not been a problem for them, their relations with doctors had been plagued by negative feelings and incidents. Interviewees raising this theme often connected the negative feelings they had toward doctors with their unwillingness to seek prompt follow-up in response to the clinic report. Several persons interviewed, for example, expressed highly critical opinions about the incomes earned by modern American physicians. Respondents produced a spate of comments in this vein, condemning physicians for their "monopoly power" and characterizing them as "rip-off artists" and "robber barons." In what can be interpreted as a reaction to the extraordinary status claims of physicians in the late twentieth century, one respondent in the face-to-face interviewing said that he disliked doctors because they "all thought they were gods."

A second theme that expressed deep unease in relationships with physicians concerned the degree to which respondents felt they could be trusted to do a good, careful job of diagnosis and treatment. Several interviewees expressed low opinions of the conscientiousness of the doctors whose services they had utilized themselves or those rendered to kin, citing specific incidents that they felt lowered their confidence in the medical profession. Comments such as, "I hate doctors . . . they don't have time to take care of you," abounded. One man expressed the suspicion that his father, stricken with cancer, died not of the disease but of "experimental drugs" that physicians had administered. A particularly articulate respondent connected her mistrust of physicians with the death of a sister that she felt could have been prevented. According to her description, the sister had died because a doctor had failed to take her symptoms seriously, and when she was finally diagnosed, she was found to have had cancer for some time. At the time of diagnosis, the sister had an extensively diffused malignancy, and she soon died.

A third opinion widely expressed among this sample of noncompliers was that physicians could really do very little to cure malignancies. These respondents often made explicit connections between their low estimation of the medical profession's ability to manage cancerous conditions and their disinclination to follow up the clinic's indications that they might have cancer. The evaluations expressed by these noncompliers ranged from incredulity about the physician's abilities vis-à-vis cancer to specification of negative utilities faced by individuals who sought treatment for malignancies. Respondents in the face-to-face procedure commented:

> I don't think the medical profession does well in general in curing and treating cancer. It's almost always fatal . . . my sister, aunt and others were all treated and died.
>
> Operations for cancer aren't that successful, my father died of cancer . . . maybe (the cure will come) for my children's children.
>
> The efforts to cure cancer are not successful today . . . and some cancer treatments can do more harm than good.
>
> They won't cure cancer . . . they just prolong death . . . they use people as guinea pigs.
>
> I don't like what I've heard about cancer treatment . . . people end up dying anyway.
>
> If I had cancer, I'd kill myself . . . I don't want to take all the money (for treatment) away from my family.

Lastly, interviewees responding in the face-to-face procedure often connected poor personal relationships they had experienced with physicians with their disinclination to follow up the Metropolitan directive. Most often, complaints about personal relations with physicians involved the distance practitioners tended to keep from patients and methods of communication perceived as inadequate. One respondent's comments touched on both themes:

I've had bad experiences with doctors. I've never found a family doctor I was satisfied with in fifteen years. The warmth is missing. I don't like to be kept in the dark . . . they're evasive.

Another expressed similar sentiments:

I insist that my family see a doctor, but I don't hold (physicians) in too high esteem. The farther people keep away from them, the better off they'll be . . . I go when I'm in pain and when my wife insists. I consider them a bunch of egotists. They conceal information from us.

A third expressed displeasure at the tendency of many practitioners he had encountered to issue only the most guarded of diagnoses:

All the doctor says is "well, it might be this, it might be that." I can do as well myself!

And, in a statement paralleling recent sociological analyses, a woman suggested:

Doctors always try to conceal information from patients. That's how they keep their power over us.

The negative association between close relations with the health care system in general and doctors in particular and delay in follow-up indicated by the multiple regression analysis is reflected in the screenees' comments. Many connect their delay or avoidance of follow-up with poor access to physicians' services, mistrust of physicians, low estimation of the doctor's ability to deal effectively with cancer, and unsatisfactory personal relations with practitioners. The statistical association between naming a family doctor and promptly following up the clinic recommendations may reflect the fact that patients who have already established access find follow-up more convenient, or that those who have sufficient confidence in doctors to procure a regular source of treatment are also the most strongly inclined to seek medical consultations at the suggestion of the clinic.

Of course, the dread associated with cancer suggests that at least some comments in the face-to-face procedure represented justification for inaction. The face-to-face interviewing included depth interviewing techniques designed to detect this process. The interviews revealed several obvious instances of justification and denial, interviewees abandoning their original explanations as the interview sessions progressed. An individual who had cited difficulty in making a doctor's appointment, for example, eventually commented, "I'm just a lazy person," and, "I'm having too much fun to go see the doctor." In extreme cases, respondents would at last admit extreme fear of the dread disease, commenting, "If I have cancer, I don't want to know about it." One older woman with a suspicious mass in her urinary tract at first offered an elaborate justification of her inaction in terms of the time costs of medical attention:

> I don't have time. I can't make time. I'd have to go to the hospital and that would take time. . . . I have to take care of my son who is sick, and I can't stop working. Maybe after I retire. . . .

But a few moments later she commented, with a show of emotion: "I know I'm ignoring this condition. I'm really very afraid."

Fear, however, seemed to play a small part in explaining delay. The multiple regression analysis above indicates a positive relation between the number of blood relatives reported to have died of cancer (a correlate of the respondent's concern with the prospects of contracting the disease) and prompt follow-up. However, the relation explains only a small portion of the variance in the time screenees take to follow up the clinic directives. The older woman with the urinary tract mass, furthermore, may have offered an accurate indication of the barriers she faced in obtaining needed care as well as expressing a very reasonable level of anxiety. A retail sales worker, this respondent may have faced serious penalties for taking off time to see a physician for a nonacute condition. Had she occupied a professional position, the necessity of taking time off to comply with the clinic recommendations might have proved less burdensome. As Yelin et al. note in rheumatic disease patients, those with high status jobs find it easier than others to take time off to see physicians.[25] And in the present study, the multiple regression analysis indicates that the higher the respondent's occupational status, the less the tendency to delay or avoid follow-up. It is noteworthy that occupational status is the only statistically significant social background variable in the analysis. This observation is not surprising since, unlike occupational status, qualities such as age and educational level imply no concrete set of structural and work authority relationships as does occupational status.

A variety of individual attitudes and attributes seem to be associated with noncompliance and delay. Both the statistical and depth-interview methods generate complementary research .findings. The analysis presented thus far, though, deals with only a few possible outcomes of interrelationships among variables and makes no attempt at determining relations that develop over time. A more detailed analysis of the face-to-face interview data helps complete the picture.

### Expectations, Motivations, and Noncompliance

The connection between the screenee's relationship with the health care system and noncompliance receives support from both the face-to-face interviews and the statistical analysis. The notion that individuals with poor access to physicians or other health care providers, or those who feel repelled from the health care system despite good access, should be the least strongly inclined to respond promptly to Metropolitan's directives is hardly a counterintuitive finding. A much more problematical and potentially important issue, however, is why individuals with these negative relations with the health care system seek care at a facility like Metropolitan in the first place. An understanding of why these persons approach the screening center generates an explanation of noncompliance on the basis of conflicts between expectations, motivations, and experiences at the clinic. While the diversity of complicated personal conflicts in this area are difficult to capture in a mathematical model, they have important implications for the behavior of groups that would be newly included in screening activities if facilities of this kind were expanded on a large scale. The joint contributions of motivations, expectations, and experiences on noncompliance generate both the most powerful explanations of the phenomenon and the clearest implications for health policy related to cancer screening.

Several different types of motivations apprently brought people to the clinic for screening. According to the face-to-face interviews, individuals seemed to seek out the clinic services as substitutes or supplements for some major aspects of primary care as it is conventionally provided in modern American society. Primary care is the most neglected feature of medical care in our society, a source of special concern for middle-class Americans, who have experienced a decline in availability of this service and frequently express the feeling that its quality has declined in recent years.[26] Briefly, our interviews detected three distinct patterns in people's motivations to seek screening at Metropolitan: increased economy and convenience in comparison with other sources of primary care, disapproval and mistrust of physicians in conventional settings, and a desire to play a more active role in their own health care. The differences that individuals with these goals perceived between their expectations and services received at Metropolitan seem to explain much noncompliant behavior.

Price, of course, is among the simplest explanations of human behavior. It plays a definite part in the decisions of individuals to visit the Metropolitan Screening Clinic over other options when they are concerned with catching threats to their health at an early stage. Many of our respondents reported that they chose Metropolitan at least partially for economic reasons. Some mentioned that the number of tests at Metropolitan would cost far more than the clinic's $80 fee if administered in a hospital, laboratory, or through a doctor's office. One respondent estimated the cost of Metropolitan's services if obtained elsewhere at $600. Even screenees who were not entranced with Metropolitan's equipment or procedure expressed appreciation of the price. As one man mentioned, "they are not *that* advanced a facility, but it's a good buy for what you get."

The individuals we interviewed expressed material advantages in Metropolitan's procedure that were nonmonetary as well. They said it was easier to get medical evaluation at the clinic than elsewhere. One respondent told us that she had not been able to find an acceptable "family" doctor for some time and went to Metropolitan as a substitute. Another interviewee said that he could get an appointment at Metropolitan in two weeks' time, which was much better than his regular doctor could do in scheduling. A third individual expressed satisfaction with the time the procedure required, noting that the screenee was "in and out" in under three hours. A fourth depicted hospitalization for a series of diagnostic tests, an alternative to the services offered by Metropolitan as "dehumanizing and disgusting." For some interviewees, attending the clinic appeared to be merely the most convenient method of obtaining primary care. "I went to the Clinic because I hadn't had a good physical in years," and "I went to Metropolitan for a physical exam; the cancer checkup wasn't that important," were some respondents' comments in this vein.

In addition to the cost and convenience features that respondents noted about the clinic, numerous comments came out about perceptions of low-quality diagnostic services in more conventional settings. Several respondents told stories about physicians who had missed important symptoms in examinations of themselves or others, tracing their motivation for attending the clinic to disappointment with the medical profession for this reason. The woman described above, whose sister's malignancy went unnoticed by a family physician and eventually led to a "preventable" death, became an avid client of Metropolitan because of this experience. Although her story was

especially striking, many other respondents in the face-to-face interviewing expressed similar sentiments and provided similar narratives.

Much evidence arose in the interviews that the desire to take
greater personal responsibility for one's health—sometimes characterized as a "self-care movement" in American society as a whole[27]—
is often an important motivational factor in drawing people to
Metropolitan. Preventive medicine, of which the clinic is an approximation, appeals to the educated, aware population that contributes most heavily to Metropolitan's caseload. Individuals transmitted
to us the feeling that because doctors were too busy or unconcerned
with their problems, they had to take active steps on their own to
assure good health, or at least the early detection of cancer. Others
expressed a feeling that they could do much of what a doctor does
for them themselves, several interviewees reporting that they pur-
chased medication or devices for themselves when possible to "avoid
the middleman." It is worth remembering that Metropolitan's population of screenees, with its high level of education, is in a better
position to evaluate the intellectual merits of physicians and more
prone to criticize physicians for not treating them as equals than the
population at large. For these critics, the mechanized structure of
the clinic offered an alternative. As one individual commented, "the
machines do a better job than the doctors . . . we live in a machine
age, anyway."

The multiphasic, automatic operation at Metropolitan appealed
directly to the desire of many screenees to contribute actively to
their own health care. Several felt they could better evaluate the
standardized, often quantitative data the tests generated than the
vague utterances of many physicians. Few indicated the feeling that
the automated procedures used at the clinic could become substitutes for "a careful examination by a competent physician." The
telephone survey revealed, for example, that the vast majority of
screenees (93 percent) rated the physician's examination at Metropolitan as valuable compared with a slightly smaller percentage (87
percent) rating the clinic's instruments as valuable. But many thought
the instruments provided clarification of their condition, which was
unusual in a doctor's office. The ability of screenees to help operate
some of the clinic's equipment also appealed to some. "You feel like
you are doing it for yourself," commented one respondent, expressing satisfaction with the self-operated, computerized health history
questionnaire.

It is clear that many clients looked upon Metropolitan as an opportunity to avoid some of the major problems they perceived in the
care they had received or could receive in other settings. For many,

the clinic was simply more accessible than other sources of diagnostic services. For others, the clinic represented an opportunity to participate more actively in at least one area of health care, that of preventive medicine. For some, this impulse to participate meant a desire to assist the physician by making more information available to him or her, for others, the desire to achieve greater equality and satisfaction by sharing diagnostic information with the physician.

Many of the noncompliers interviewed in the face-to-face procedure traced their behavior to disappointment with the clinic, contrasting actual experiences with initial expectations. Several individuals who had clearly come to Metropolitan in search of medical care of a type unavailable in the wider system found the clinic wanting. One screenee who had indicated a desire for a clear, honest diagnosis as a reason for visiting the clinic reported extreme disappointment with the letter she received from Metropolitan. Perhaps misunderstanding the distinction between "diagnosis" and "screening," this client found the clinic's letter informing her only that her test results had indicated a "missing enzyme" a disappointment. Another, visiting the clinic in hopes of obtaining knowledge about a highly visible growth on his nose, expressed both surprise and dismay at the directive from Metropolitan to "see a doctor." Still others interviewed face-to-face noted that they had visited the clinic in order to obtain more careful examinations than they felt they could receive in a doctor's office, but felt extreme disappointment when clinic personnel either did not notice or spend much time examining the symptom that motivated them to come. Lastly, individuals who came to Metropolitan either for a more participatory form of medical care or for more "humane" treatment than they had experienced in the health care system as a whole reported unrealized expectations. Some individuals in this category traced their noncompliant behavior to the automated features of the clinic procedure. Apparently, this characteristic of Metropolitan led to the disappointment and noncompliance of several individuals surveyed in the face-to-face interviews. "You're like an object going down an assembly line," and "I felt just like a slab of meat," commented two of these noncompliers.

For some individuals, the unexpected task of moving independently from the clinic to providers of actual diagnostic and therapeutic services proved too great. Some felt that they had already spent as much money on cancer detection as they felt necessary, evincing a strong disinclination to expend further resources for this purpose. The individual who looked to Metropolitan for convenience, for example, seemed to feel overburdened by the necessity of going farther in the health care system when the clinic indicated this was necessary. The screenee with the nose lesion provides a case in point. He apparently approached the clinic with the expectation of a quick, clear *on-site* diagnosis of this visible problem. The role of this screenee's expectations about the clinic is particularly clear in the light of his compliance behavior in response to directives from Metropolitan and from a practitioner in a more conventional setting:

> I went to Metropolitan for convenience . . . someone in the office told me I should go because of my family's (cancer) history . . . I was disappointed because the clinic would not diagnose the sore on my nose . . . they told me to see a doctor . . . you don't spend eighty bucks to have them tell you to see a specialist . . . they should have diagnosed it . . . I did eventually follow up (on the problem) after my son's eye doctor told me to see a specialist "right away."

Those whose expectations were apparently contradicted by the clinic often focused on the affective content of the communications rather than their factual content. The screenee with the nose problem explained part of his willingness to see a specialist as his personal relation with the physician who recommended this action. Although this physician did not even examine the screenee, an affective element of his relationship with the screenee played an important part in his decision to finally seek medical follow-up. The screenee explained that he at last followed up because this doctor "had my confidence" and "showed concern." Others indicated additional connections between their compliance behavior and the emotive content of communications from the clinic. A woman directed to follow up a positive mammogram told the interviewer:

> I didn't get alarmed, the breast lump has been there for a long time . . . they didn't give me a diagnosis . . . they just told me to check it out . . . but that was why I went there. Without a diagnosis, it's not important enough to go (to a follow-up).

Others, either taking the indefinite nature of the clinic communications as a genuine indication that no serious condition existed or using the associated ambiguity as an excuse to justify inaction, connected the lack of specificity and urgency in Metropolitan's letters with their inaction. The connection between lack of urgency and noncompliance with the Metropolitan directives occurred repeatedly:

> I knew about by problem before . . . (there was) no sense of emergency generated by the letter . . . if they had set out some of the things that

might happen to you . . . it might frighten people into the doctor's office . . . that's fine.

It it were serious I would go to a doctor . . . my family would not let me do nothing (in that case).

The letter really didn't affect me . . . the doctor didn't indicate much concern.

It was generally apparent in the face-to-face interviews that individuals who expected contact with the clinic to involve minimal difficulties tended to avoid medical follow-up when informed of positive findings. Several of the noncompliers interviewed, for example, reported feelings that they were in good health before attending the clinic, and when informed of suspicious findings, they were unwilling to change their minds. Concrete test results were not always sufficient to convince such screenees otherwise. As one screenee told the interviewer:

I went to the screening because it was free for all of us at work . . . I did not feel the tests were valid . . . a technician threw away a sample of my blood . . . I'm not sure that it was a sample of my blood that was tested . . . there must be some mix-up . . . (the findings were) irrelevant, invalid and an illusion . . . I may be sick but I doubt it . . . I'm not concerned, I don't feel sick . . . there are no signs . . . (I would go back) if they would show me that the test results were valid and mine . . . not until then.

The gap between the screenee's expectation of a nonproblematical encounter with the health care system through Metropolitan and actual experiences involving, at best, inconvenience, and, at worst, extreme fear of illness and death seems to explain the noncompliant behavior of many individuals in the face-to-face interviews. One of the best examples of this gap in expectations and experiences seems to occur among those who attend the clinic at the persuasion of others. Those whose personal motivations are insufficient to bring them to Metropolitan, for instance, would express greater sensitivity to inconvenience than others. One woman explained:

I usually skip my appointments with doctors . . . my mother (who had cancer) wanted me to have my breasts checked . . . so I went to Metropolitan . . . I still don't believe anything is wrong, even though I haven't been back to see anything about it . . . I think they should recommend a follow-up doctor . . . I might have gone then.

For individuals whose visit to Metropolitan was not completely self-motivated, noncompliance seemed to accompany lack of continuing social support. Thus, the company or persuasion of others might be sufficient to bring a screenee to the clinic doors, but insufficient in strength or duration to motivate compliance with directives to seek medical follow-up. Another woman's comments illustrate this scenario:

> I have a girl friend who went with me during working hours . . . our boss let us go, he gave us time off after another lady at work told us about the place . . . the doctor (at the clinic) said I should get them (skin lesions) off . . . she (her girl friend) has warts that she was told to have off . . . she says that she'll go (to the doctor) if I go . . . she's always bugging me . . . as a matter of fact, we both made an appointment . . . but one of us couldn't make it, so we both canceled . . . and we never made it back again . . . if they (the clinic doctors) had said it would mean cancer, I would have gone . . . but they didn't, and (the skin lesions) don't hurt me.

Screenees with suspicious findings, however, provided examples of follow-up behavior in response to encouragement from others for whom they had great respect or long-lasting, intimate relations. The screenee with the nose lesion fell into this category. Attributing his decision to eventually follow up his clinic visit to the influence of his son's ophthalmologist and his wife, he commented:

> I have confidence in that doctor. He showed concern . . . My wife kept insisting too, and I think that reinforced (the doctor's urging).

Among many Metropolitan screenees, strong disparities seem to occur between expectations and experiences. Some individuals expect the clinic to reassure them that they are in good health and are unwilling to make the sacrifices necessary when findings indicate otherwise. Other screenees identified as noncompliers appear to expect continuing support from friends, co-workers, or physicians to take the necessary action in response to positive findings, only to find this support nonexistent or weaker than anticipated. Still others seek to remedy shortcomings in the wider health care system by visiting Metropolitan and find the clinic unable to provide what they seek.

The effect of the attitude with which the screenee approaches Metropolitan on the tendency to comply with its directives is highly consistent with the statistical analysis presented above. As Table 7-7 indicates, persons with middle-level commitments to "periodic, routine physicals to maintain good health" appear to be the most likely to delay. Many of these individuals, with middle-level commitments to processes akin to screening at Metropolitan, may have attended the clinic in response to "peripheral" motivators such as convenience, economy, or persuasion by others. Screenees approaching the clinic for these reasons appear to have relatively weak commitments to follow up, either because they are unwilling to undertake the difficult and fear-arousing action related to cancer diagnosis or because they are fundamentally unconcerned with preventive health care behavior. In contrast, those with strong commitments to periodic examinations tend to comply promptly. Those with especially *weak* commitments to periodic, routine examinations also seem to comply promptly with Metropolitan's directives. This finding is surprising at first, but it takes on meaning when viewed in the light of Table 7-4. This table indicates that those with low commitments to periodic examinations are significantly more likely to appear at the clinic in response to visible symptoms than others, or to be referred there by physicians. While uncommitted to periodic, routine physicals, many of these individuals may have additional motivations to comply: the visible presence of symptoms and the legitimacy imparted to the screening process by referring physicians.

## THE PROBLEM OF DELAY

This chapter has touched upon two major problems related to the efficacy of cancer screening, problems that will persist even if the technology of early detection is improved to an extraordinary degree of perfection. The literature on preventive health care behavior strongly suggests that cancer detection facilities will be utilized primarily by an "elite" of educated, white, and otherwise socially advantaged people. Tentative observations of the Metropolitan Screening Clinic suggest that this is indeed the case. The literature on health services also suggests that many problems should arise for cancer screening in compliance. Again, this chapter demonstrates that such problems do exist for the Metropolitan Screening Clinic. While this chapter does not address the issue of differential utilization directly, it does provide planners and scholars with a detailed explanation of why even an elite clientele should harbor numerous noncompliers.

The factors affecting noncompliance with the Metropolitan recommendations for medical follow-up strongly resemble those observed by researchers in several other contexts. The face-to-face interviews reported here, for example, clearly indicate that many noncompliers express feelings of invulnerability. The multiple regression analysis supports this observation, providing evidence that some individuals whose family histories are free from cancer deaths view the clinic findings with less urgency than those with relatives who died of cancer. These findings are quite similar to those reported by Becker and Maiman[28] and Hochbaum[29] linking perceived danger of illness to seeking helath care.

As reported in other contexts, the quality of communication between physician and patient appears quite important in promoting or discouraging follow-up among Metropolitan screenees. The physician often plays an important though inadvert part in facilitating the screenee's process of denial. A large proportion of noncompliers reported that physicians at Metropolitan told them of a finding but either stated or implied that it was not serious. Many screenees ignored the subsequent letters from the clinic advising medical follow-up. In some cases, it was apparent that Metropolitan was sending out warnings about conditions that were medically "trivial." But it seemed certain in others that the screenee, seeking to minimize the seriousness of a finding, seized upon any comment the physician made to ease his or her mind and justify inaction.

The most important predictors of prompt follow-up at Metropolitan, however, are strong connections with other parts of the health care system. As cited above, numerous researchers report analogous phenomena in other areas of medical care: regular use of health care resources, access to care, trust of physicians, and belief in medical technology coincide with prompt approach and compliance. Both the present study and many other investigations convincingly suggest that the major explanation of delay and noncompliance in early detection efforts lies in the individual's physical and attitudinal connection with the health care system as a whole. These similarities are expecially striking in view of the differences suggested by some investigators between illness behavior related to cancer and other diseases. These findings confirm R. Fink's observation in one of the few previous studies of factors affecting follow-up in cancer screening[30] that regular use of health services correlates positively with prompt patient response to positive findings.

Systematic research on access to health care suggests a specific mechanism that may explain much of the noncompliance observed in this study. Aday and Andersen report that individuals with the poorest access to regular medical care—those with no regular doctor or who are forced to wait long periods of time before being seen—tend to be the least satisfied with medical care.[31] These dissatisfied individuals appear the least likely to seek medical care when in need.

Similarly dissatisfied individuals among Metropolitan screenees seem likely to ignore its directives. The tendency to avoid compliance would be especially severe among those who seek screening at Metropolitan as an alternative to diagnostic services that they perceive as inadequate in the regular health care system. When these screenees find that Metropolitan does not provide the quick, comprehensible diagnosis or personal attention they seek, they become even less likely to seek care in the wider system. Screenees caught up in this cycle of dissatisfaction with the health care system, disappointment with the Metropolitan Screening Clinic, and reinforced dissatisfaction with health care in general appear to be the best candidates for noncompliance. Conversely, those with strong preexisting connections with the health care system and positive attitudes toward it seem to move promptly from early detection to points of more definitive diagnosis.

It is worth noting in conclusion that fear of dread disease did not appear to play an overwhelmingly powerful role in determining delay and avoidance of medical follow-up in cancer screening. It is, of course, obvious that the threat of cancer does produce extreme fear. But the screenees interviewed in the research reported here—both derived from the face-to-face interviews and the telephone survey—indicate that many separate factors play significant roles in bringing patients to sources of definitive care or keeping them away. Screenees faced with positive findings in the present study do comply with the clinic directives in the majority of instances. Doubtlessly, many of these compliers experience fear in the process. According to the analysis presented here, though, the persons most likely to comply in short order with the clinic directives receive encouragement of some concrete kind to do so. The ready availability of regular medical care, for example, seems likely to permit individuals with suspicious findings to move easily from the screening center to a doctor's office. Access to medical care, then, seems to mean one less barrier that may deter individuals from seeking follow-up care or excuse to permit the especially fearful to avoid confronting their difficulty. The encouragement by familiar or esteemed others plays an important part in encouraging prompt compliance as well, poor doctor-patient communication promoting noncompliance not merely because information is not transmitted, but also because emotional support is not offered. The occupant of a prestigious occupation is unlikely to fear cancer less intensely than his or her blue-collar counterpart. The prestigious jobholder, though, must make fewer demands on his or her skills to maneuver through a highly fragmented health care system—the fragmentation of which is amply demonstrated by the gaps between Metropolitan and other health care facilities—than the individual in a lower status job. While fear is always present, social structural features of the individual's situation play an important part in the ability to actively confront the threatening situation. The findings here recall research by Shils and Janowitz demonstrating that soldiers in a defeated army continued to fight as long as their primary groups survived, encouraging individuals to carry on despite discouraging odds.[32] Constructing analogous social supports may improve the compliance rate in cancer detection. This necessity, as well as the forging of more reliable linkages between early detection and actual diagnostic and treatment sites, seems certain to become even more important in screening efforts directed at populations less consistently inclined to seek early detection than the elite of preventive health care seekers studied here. Thus, the social factor is crucial in the successful implementation of the mandate of the National Cancer Act for early detection.

Analysts should view the issue of noncompliance in cancer screening not merely as a product of individual personality characteristics and the general public's fear of cancer, but as an outcome of the health care system's arrangements for providing screening services. Central features of the social technology now in use among health care providers in the cancer control program service region clearly contribute to noncompliance, making a key goal in cancer control more remote. Recall from Chapter 2 that control of cancer as well as all modern diseases requires methods quite different from those that conquered infectious ailments. Among the most important factors that this chapter argues are necessary for control of modern disease, three seem especially important in improving the efficacy of screening on a regionwide basis. They are (1) increased initiative by health care providers to reach individuals who can benefit from screening and other preventive measures; (2) better integration of the health care system to meet the multifaceted needs of modern disease sufferers more efficiently; and (3) more emphasis on emotional support to encourage the patient during lengthy and discouraging periods of treatment. Deficiencies on all these dimensions appear to contribute to the noncompliance problem at the Metropolitan Screening Clinic. Because clients seek out the clinic on a largely random and voluntary basis, the screenee population reflects a very specific segment of the area's residents. Because the automated procedures of the clinic provide no personal encouragement for screenees to overcome very reasonable fears of cancer, many succumb to the natural tendency to avoid seeking conclusive diagnosis and treatment. Because the clinic maintains no well-established linkages with organizations providing health care of a different but complementary nature, screenees often become discouraged in their search for follow-up care. If asymptomatic screening is typical of other cancer-related health services, basic revisions in the social technology surrounding such activities must accompany innovations in medical technology to appreciably reduce morbidity and mortality from cancer. Chapter 8 suggests some starting points in this complex and difficult task.

## NOTES

1. D.J. Fink, "The Cancer Control Program." *Cancer* 35 (1975): 72-75.

2. D.G. Miller, "What Is Early Detection Doing?" *Cancer* 37 (1976): 426-432.

3. Ibid., p. 427.

4. D. Colburn, and C.R. Pope, "Socioeconomic Status and Preventive Health Behavior." *Journal of Health and Social Behavior* 15 (1974): 67-78.

5. B. Kutner and G. Gordon et al., "Seeking Care for Cancer." *Journal of Health and Human Behavior* 2 (Fall 1961): 171-178.

6. R. Fink, "Delay Behavior in Breast Cancer Screening," in J.W. Cullen et al., eds., *Cancer: The Behavioral Dimension* (New York: Raven Press, 1976); pp. 19-33.

7. H.B. Makover, "Patient and Physician Delay in Cancer Diagnosis: Medical Aspects," *Journal of Chronic Disease* 16 (1963): 419-426.

8. G.T. Pack, and J.S. Gallo, "Culpability for Delay in Treatment of Cancer," *American Journal of Cancer* 33 (1938): 443-462.

9. H.B. Makover, op. cit.

10. F.H. Rodenbough, "Multiphasic Screening Makes Me Sick," *Medical Economics* 13 (September 1973): 6-12.

11. S.M. Shortell and O.W. Anderson, "The Physician Referral Process: A Theoretical Perspective," *Health Services Research* 21 (Spring 1971): 39-48.

12. T. Parsen, *The Social System* (Glencoe, Ill: The Free Press, 1951). See Chapter 10.

13. E. Koos, *The Health of Regionsville: What People Thought and Did About It* (New York: Columbia University Press, 1954).

14. E.A. Suchman, "Stages of Illness and Medical Care," *Journal of Health and Human Behavior* 6 (1965): 114-128.

15. D. Mechanic, *Medical Sociology* (New York: The Free Press, 1968). See p. 131.

16. R. Andersen, *A Behavioral Model of Families' Use of Health Services* (Chicago: Center for Health Administration Studies, Research Series No. 25, 1968).

17. L.A. Aday, "Economic and Noneconomic Barriers to the Use of Needed Medical Services," *Medical Care* 13 (June 1975): 467-456. See p. 453.

18. H.M. Becker and L.A. Maiman, "Sociobehavioral Determinants of Com-

pliance with Health Care Recommendations," *Medical Care* 13 (January 1975): 11-24.

19. R.M. Batistella, "Factors Associated with Delay in the Initiation of Physicians' Care among Late Adulthood Persons," *American Journal of Public Health* 61 (1971): 1348.

20. B.M. Korsch et al., "Gaps in Doctor-Patient Communication I: Doctor-Patient Satisfaction," *Pediatrics* 42 (1968): 885-871.

21. M.S. Davis, "Discharge from Hospitals Against Medical Advice: A Study of Reciprocity in the Doctor-Patient Relationship," *Social Science and Medicine* 1 (1960): 336-344.

22. E. Chauney, "How Well Do Patients Take Oral Penicillin: A Collaborative Study in Private Practice," *Pediatrics* 40 (1967): 188-195.

23. B. Cobb et al., "Patient Responsible Delay in Treatment of Cancer," *Cancer* 7 (September, 1954): 920-925. See also Kutner and Gordon, op. cit.

24. P. Blau and O.D. Duncan, *The American Occupational Structure* (New York: John Wiley, 1967).

25. E.H. Yelin et al. "Social Problems, Services, and Policy for Persons with Rheumatoid Arthritis," *Social Science and Medicine* 13C (March, 1979): 13-20.

26. R. Andersen, J. Kravits, and D.W. Anderson, "The Public's View of the Crisis in Medical Care: An Impetus for Changing Delivery Systems?" *Economic and Business Bulletin* 24 (Fall 1971): 44-52.

27. Gretchen V. Fleming and Ronald Anderson, *Health Beliefs of the U.S. Population: Implications for Self-Care* (Chicago: University of Chicago Center for Health Administration Studies, 1977).

28. Becker and Maiman, op. cit.

29. G.M. Hochbaum, *Public Participation in Medical Screening Programs: A Socio-psychological Study* (Washington, D.C.: U.S. Government Printing Office, Public Health Service Publication No. 572, 1958).

30. Fink, op. cit.

31. L.A. Aday and R. Andersen, *Access to Medical Care* (Ann Arbor, Mich.: Health Administration Press, 1975), pp. 75-76.

32. E.A. Shils and M. Janowitz, "Cohesion and Disintegration in the Wehrmacht in World War II," *Public Opinion Quarterly* 12 (1948): 280-315.

# Chapter 8

# Conclusion: Public Policy and Cancer Control

The preceding chapters suggest several important short-comings in the capacity of health care providers in the cancer control program service region to combat malignancies in the systematic, coordinated, and comprehensive manner proposed by the National Cancer Act of 1971. Some shortcomings visible in the region's cancer-fighting activities stem from an imbalance of resources. As Chapter 3 reports, the cancer control program service region appeared to have an adequate supply of material resources, including hospital beds and high technology equipment for cancer diagnosis and therapy. The region, however, seemed to lack sufficient professional personnel in appropriate specialties, a comprehensive network of early detection centers, and reliable sources of emotional support for cancer patients and their families. Many of the physical facilities and professional practices in the region were located at sites inconvenient for large numbers of the area residents, a situation aggravated by inadequate transportation. Relations among health care professionals and organizations appeared to present difficulties at least as important as the availability of resources. The prevailing pattern of professional relationships, for example, seemed inconducive to an efficient flow of information on new cancer-related techniques from the university medical center to community practitioners. Long-established professional predilections and networks seemed capable of blocking the movement of patients to potentially lifesaving sources of secondary and tertiary care. Patterns of day-to-day interaction between physicians and nurses seemed to discourage nurses from including emotional support for cancer patients as part of their work routines.

Difficulties of this nature suggest that improved control of cancer requires the development of a new social technology in health care, a system of interpersonal and interorganizational relations that enables the public to receive the full benefits of laboratory and clinical research more reliably than in the current system. A vigorous community of physicians whose norms, values, and rewards encourage the continuous exchange of knowledge and patients and sharing of responsibilities for patient care is a key element of this social technology. The new social technology also requires more willing delegation of important responsibilities to nurses and other non-physician health professionals and more active encouragement of individuals in the community to seek early detection and treatment of malignancies. Those who sought to promote this new social technology in the cancer control program service region made valuable progress among forward-looking professionals and within particularly cooperative hospitals and clinics. But their efforts encountered serious barriers in the form of practices that prevailed among health care providers throughout the United States and special difficulties related to the university medical center's traditional place in the local community.

This concluding chapter has a twofold objective: first, to link the findings presented here about cancer to broader, continuing issues in contemporary health planning and policy and, second, to offer concrete suggestions to individuals in planning roles concerned with the control of any modern disease. Containing both pessimistic and optimistic features, this dual approach runs two complementary risks of misleading readers. Some, for example, may feel that concrete strategies such as those presented below exhaust the capacity of modern society to control cancer given existing levels of scientific and medical understanding. This is not the case. Immediate strategies leave many large-scale issues untouched whose resolution is a definite precondition for optimal cancer control in modern American society. Other readers may consider immediate strategies trivial, arguing that only basic changes in the entire health care system, if not contemporary society in general, will significantly reduce the threat that cancer represents to life and the quality of living. Even if fundamentally true, this argument would not render immediate planning strategies meaningless. As noted at the beginning of this book, even a slight reduction of the death rate from a disease as widespread as cancer may mean additional years of life for numerous individuals. Improvement in the quality of life for a small proportion of cancer sufferers may transform debilitating conditions into tolerable ones for many. This concluding discussion strives to help planners do as much as possible within existing frameworks for health care delivery while remembering that successful applications of immediate strategies still leave questions of the highest importance unanswered.

In line with the general approach of this investigation, the discussion of concrete strategies and general issues does not attempt to be exhaustive. Numerous, important considerations remain untouched, such as the cost-benefit issues implied by various features of cancer control and the question of community participation in regional health planning. These issues are no less significant than those on which the current investigation focuses. Other researchers concerned with cancer control or similar health policy areas can make important contributions by providing insights into these matters. The present volume intends to provide a limited range of material to illustrate the importance of social relations in inhibiting or promoting effective cancer detection and treatment on a regionally coordinated basis. Rather than a set of principles immediately applicable in all localities, it illustrates the *type* of concrete approach that planners in numerous geographical locations are likely to find useful.

The discussion to follow casts both policy issues and immediate strategies as dilemmas. Resolution of the major, macrosocial issues raised here will require years of continuing exploration and debate. Arising from both accidents of history and essential features of medical practice everywhere in the modern world, large-scale policy issues related to cancer control cannot be approached effectively through simple theories or social dogma. Application of immediate strategies for the small-scale improvement of cancer control will take place in a similar atmosphere of uncertainty and experimentation. This chapter's suggestions are not formulas but possible approaches for individuals willing to confront suspicion and resistance. Though intellectually and politically unsatisfying to some, this approach may be the most reasonable not only for cancer control or health care, but also for any major policy issue.

## CANCER CONTROL AND GENERAL POLICY ISSUES

Among the major social problems involved in cancer control, the most important may involve the limits that existing patterns of power and resource allocation in the overall health care system place upon innovation. Often, this arrangement of power and resources seems to contradict society's attempt to meet needs associated with the diseases that constitute today's major health concerns. Patients with modern diseases require continuity of care from provider to provider, access to high technology equipment located at only a few hospitals in any given region, the benefits of recently developed therapeutic techniques, and a variety of support services. Just as the preceding investigation has identified widespread inability to meet these requirements in cancer, investigators of other attempts to re-organize health care have reported similar inadequacies and resistance to change. The discussion to follow treats only two sources of these inadequacies, the lack of coordination among health care providers and the inability of nonphysician health professionals to fully utilize their capacities. These issues, however, only illustrate what is perhaps the most difficult problem in providing more effective control of cancer: existing patterns of power and dominance.

One major concept that exposes the problems associated with power and resource allocation is that of "regionalization." Appearing in legislation as early as the Hill-Burton Act, regionalization provisions call for linkages among health care providers of higher and lower capacity "so that patients who enter the health system at the periphery have access to the complete spectrum of services through prearranged channels."[1] In an important review article on the Regional Medical Program instituted under PL89-239 in 1965, Bodenheimer lists four mechanisms by which policymakers hoped to bring about regional coordination among providers:

> These linkages fall into four categories—the referral of patients from peripheral to central institutions, the back-and-forth flow of patient records, consultation by specialists from central to peripheral institutions, and continuing education from central to peripheral institutions.[2]

While the legislation originally connected regionalization with the needs of cancer, heart disease, and stroke victims, it reflected a general sentiment among health policymakers that the American public needed a better coordinated system of health care.

Analysts cannot help but view the cancer control provisions of the National Cancer Act as a restatement of the need for regionalization. But the new call for regional coordination among health care providers appears to have encountered the same difficulties that confronted the Regional Medical Program. As Chapter 4 indicates, physicians in the cancer control program service region often viewed the university medical center's outreach program as a threat to their autonomy. They argued that they needed no assistance from the university, and they hinted that cooperation with the program would cost them patients, as individuals referred to the university medical center never returned to the care of their original physicians. Interviews with community physicians clearly suggested that many interpreted the university's invitation to participate in a regionally coordinated effort to control cancer as at best a status threat, and at worst, a threat to their incomes and the economic viability of the hospitals at which they practiced.

In his examination of the Regional Medical Program, Bodenheimer reports strikingly similar resistance to earlier attempts at regionalization of health care. Citing an extensive literature, he enumerates several major reasons why health care providers typically resist regionalization, whatever its specific disease focus. He notes, for example, that hospitals usually value their autonomy more than the financial incentives government can provide to encourage coordination and sharing of resources. In a formulation clearly reflecting the situation observed at the university medical center, he writes that medical schools, around which regionalization efforts are often organized, often avoid making serious commitments to the effort for fear of diluting their commitment to research and teaching. Physicians, of course, have both economic and ideological disincentives to refer patients to other practitioners. Implicit in this formulation is a disincentive particularly troublesome for cancer control, which depends on the willingness of community physicians to refer patients with nonroutine complaints to more specialized doctors. It seems likely that the ability to handle these cases is especially prized by local physicians. Quoting Eli Ginzberg, Bodenheimer writes:

> The success of any system (of coordinated hospital service) depends in the first instance upon the cooperation of the local physicians, whose cooperation can be secured only if they are convinced that the plan will aid them professionally and that their economic position will not be jeopardized through loss of their more interesting and difficult cases.[3]

Resistance from organizations representing various categories of professionals in health care also played an important part in rendering the Regional Medical Program's efforts ineffective. The American Medical Association, for example, lobbied powerfully with President Johnson and Secretary of Health, Education, and Welfare Gardner for a highly voluntaristic wording of the legislation and dominance of physicians on governing boards of specific regional programs. The AMA also fought for weaker linkages among health care providers than the initiators of the legislation had initially proposed. These included the requirement that patients had to be referred to university medical centers through their own physicians. But the AMA alone cannot be blamed for the weak linkage mechanisms that characterized the Regional Medical Program. According to Bodenheimer, local health departments also discouraged regionalization, since they viewed their mandate as seeking solutions to health problems on a local rather than a regional basis. In general, Bodenheimer concludes that different sets of values and interests held by the institutions that compose the U.S. health care system constitute great barriers to cooperation.[4]

The striking similarity of Bodenheimer's analysis of the Regional Medical Program and the present volume's characterization of cancer control suggests that little has changed in the intervening years. Regionalization contradicts basic desires of providers to protect their autonomy and interests. Similar factors account for the reluctance of many physicians in the cancer control program service region to refer patients to the university medical center. An exaggerated sense of pluralism, then, is one of the basic institutional features of the contemporary health care system that makes it inhospitable to the aims of the cancer control program and similar initiatives that contain provisions for regional coordination.

Alford provides an analytical framework that explains much of the resistance that cancer control and other regionally based programs have faced. This framework conceives of "structural interests," which are "served or not served by the way they 'fit' into the basic logic and principles by which the institutions of the society operate."[5] In many ways, the basic institutional arrangements that govern health care serve the interests of the community physician and community hospital, as opposed to demands for regionalization. The strength of the basic institutional arrangements governing health care manifests itself clearly in the wording of an important clause in PL 89-239, which directed the Regional Medical Program to accomplish its ends "without interfering with the patterns, or the methods of financing, of patient care or professional practice."[6]

Concretely observable features of the institutions governing health care in the contemporary United States also militate against regionalization. Prevailing methods of financing the operations of important health-related organizations provide a compelling example, with the Regional Medical Program chronically receiving too little money to initiate major local efforts[7] and hospitals, medical schools, and local health departments uninterested in regionalization easily able to obtain funding from other government agencies. The same difficulties have clearly faced organizers of cancer control programs. Medical schools that develop no major commitment to cancer control, for example, have hardly suffered as a result. These organizations still receive the bulk of their federal funding for the purpose of conducting biomedical research, and the agencies that grant funds for this purpose typically evince no interest in health services. A medical school that took cancer control seriously, furthermore, would encounter serious difficulties in maintaining its commitment. While Congress has recently shifted its attention from the laboratory to the doctor's office, administrators and grantsmen have no guarantee that this is not just a passing fad. Because of the society's long-term commitment to research, university medical centers are simply on safer ground in committing organizational resources in this direction.

Of course, regionalization is only one component of cancer control. A second important element that receives major emphasis in the preceding investigation is the need to place nonphysician medical personnel in more important roles related to cancer detection and therapy. Chapter 1, for example, details the efforts of the cancer control program to train nurses as specialists in the administration of chemotherapy and to better enable them to meet the patient's emotional needs. Chapter 3 suggests that nurses might occupy another important role, aiding in cancer screening operations in lieu of scarce primary care physicians. But as Chapter 5 points out, nurses in the cancer control program service region often feel unable to initiate contact with physicians or take needed action because of the patterns of authority that prevail in their work situations. As in its attempt to regionalize one area of health care, the efforts of the cancer control program encounter barriers related to strongly established institutional patterns.

The problems that nurses face in providing cancer patients with the services they need arise in large part from the strongly institutionalized dominance that physicians exert over all other health-related professions. The effects of this dominance on the day-to-day working relationships among physicians and nurses are well documented by Anselm Strauss. Tracing the history of the nursing profession to its nineteenth-century beginnings, Strauss identifies a fundamental duality in the nursing role. While the nurse is trained to be compassionate and humane, she also receives instruction to obey the physician's directives in the service of effective application of medical science and technology.[8] Based on their superior knowledge of this technology, physicians usually command the undisputed respect of other health professionals. In providing emotional support for patients, though, this clear line of authority tends to break down. Strauss notes that nurses are "not beholden to medical authority" for the psychological aspects of bedside nursing[9] and that serious illness and the approach of death add an element of uncertainty and disruption to working relationships on hospital wards.[10] These interruptions in the medical authority system allow nurses to exercise the emotional support capacities that play so important a part in their professional ideology. But, as noted in the present investigation, nurses often feel reluctant to take initiatives in more technical features of patient care, and they often feel they *should not* assume as important a role as they do in emotional support. Costs to the patient that arise from the authority system in health care and the nurse's ambivalent responses to it include less immediate responses from physicians to whom many nurses are afraid to make suggestions and the omission of help in adjusting emotionally to cancer. Costs to the health care system include high rates of turnover, as idealistic nurses leave the profession in search of more satisfying ways of life.

The regional planner can exert only a limited influence on the ability of health care providers to improve cancer control. Strongly institutionalized patterns of authority and resource allocation shape the basic mechanisms by which health care is offered in any given locality. Regionalization of health care can come about only if existing power relationships are altered through policy decisions at the highest level or through vocal public demands for change. Sharing of initiative among health-related professionals cannot take place before the advent of major shifts in public policy governing the training and licensure of "auxiliaries." Added to the crucial issues of industrial and environmental carcinogenesis, these factors leave the regional planner with only a narrow space for effective maneuvering. But, as noted above, cancer poses such a serious problem in modern society that even small contributions to its control are meaningful. Creative planners have initiated courses of action that have improved regional capacities to perform activites directly relevant to cancer control, and the potential exists for more such initiatives. As this volume noted at the beginning, everybody who participates in the health care system is a planner in some sense. Moves to promote control of cancer and similar health problems can originate in quarters that do not directly dispense health care but can strongly influence its method of delivery.

## IMMEDIATE STRATEGIES FOR CHANGE

Despite the limitations that face planners in any given region, many categories of people with genuine commitments to cancer control and other innovations directed at meeting needs associated with modern disease can make important contributions. Once again, individuals occupying many roles related directly or indirectly to health care can contribute to the development of the social technology necessary for more effective control of cancer. This discussion considers actions that have been taken in the past or that might be taken in the future by four categories of health-related personnel: professional health planners, hospital administrators, executives in the insurance industry, and health professionals themselves.

### Professional Health Planners

More than any other role, that of the professional health planner has an explicit connection with improved health services on a retional level. Many health planners today work for Health Systems Agencies, an organization with both planning and regulatory powers. Among analysts of the health care system, pessimism has prevailed about the potential contributions of health systems agencies for making significant changes in health care delivery. Typically, analysts consider the health systems agency powerless against the well-organized providers and, even with the aid of certificate of need legislation, able to do little other than limit further growth of an already overdeveloped sector. Wildavsky, for example, argues that the certificate of need laws will either discourage improvements in the system or increase already widespread duplication of services. "Every innovation that challenges existing interests will be attacked as unnecessary or added on to maintain harmony," he writes.[11]

This is not necessarily true. A conscientious planner associated with the health systems agency can, with detailed knowledge of the particular locality and sufficient imagination, devise mechanisms to promote the sharing of resources and cooperation among physicians that is an integral component of cancer control and similar enterprises. An example of a successful endeavor of this nature is provided by a planner for a San Francisco Bay Area health systems agency. A Kaiser-affiliated hospital in Redwood City, California, applied for a certificate of need to acquire a cardiac surgery unit. Direct opposition to this request by the health systems agency would probably have failed, given the political resources of the Kaiser system. Instead, the planner negotiated an alternative plan that gave Kaiser personnel the privilege to operate at the extensive facilities maintained at the nearby Stanford University Medical Center.

How was such a seemingly unlikely compromise accomplished? The planner knew that many of the cardiac surgeons who pushed Kaiser to acquire the new unit were graduates of the Stanford University Medical Center. These physicians would have preferred privileges at the Stanford facility but had not received positions there. At the same time, physicians at Stanford realized that the Redwood City facility, if permitted to open, would mean considerable competition in their immediate locale from physicians with qualifications and training similar to their own. Anxious to avoid competition of this kind (which would have denied the Stanford Medical Center a significant source of revenue), the Stanford faculty agreed to share its cardiac surgery facilities with Kaiser. The planner who brought about this unusual instance of cooperation possessed not only talent in negotiation but also a detailed understanding of the desires and fears of local health care providers. Planners elsewhere can benefit from applying similar techniques.

While cardiac surgery facilities are similar to cancer-related installations in cost and degree of specialization, planners interested in cancer control can apply the same negotiating technique directly to cancer. Chapter 7 strongly suggests advantages to locating screening services on the premises of hospitals, health maintenance organizations, and other organizations offering more comprehensive health services. The proximity of diagnostic and treatment services to the screening activity would reduce the difficulty of moving patients from point to point in the system; in the absence of physical proximity, strong organizational linkages would perform the same function. Planners could discourage free-standing screening facilities such as Metropolitan from maintaining too much independence by promoting relationships with hospitals or health maintenance organizations. Hospitals could be induced to cooperate in such ventures as a means of increasing in- and outpatient admissions; screening centers could use hospital clinics as sources of screenees. An able planner would be alert to specific needs of local organizations that might be articulated to the advantage of cancer control.

### Hospital Administrators

Hospital administrators often exercise planning functions. Obvious activities of this kind include purchasing and mapping out additions to the existing physical plant. The hospital administrator's scope may extend to activities closely analogous to regionalization. Administrators at a university-affiliated medical center in Pittsburgh made several seemingly effective moves to maximize the quality of their relations with the surrounding medical community. Unlike the Central City University Medical Center, the Pittsburgh facility committed a significant number of staff hours to reporting to referring physicians on the treatment their patients had received and encouraged hospital-based specialists to return the patient to the original physician's care as soon as possible. The medical center at

UCLA has a similar policy and enjoys a good reputation among referring physicians. The Pittsburgh facility, moreover, has developed a program for encouraging young physicians to open practices in the surrounding community by paying for them to open offices. According to an administrator at this hospital, the physicians maintain relations with specialists at the hospital that are valued on both sides. The community-based physician receives professional stimulation and prestige. The specialist receives increased referrals. The goal, though similar to the community outreach effort of the cancer control program, is apparently more successful at the Pittsburgh facility, where it receives more organizational resources and is pursued in a more aggressive manner.

Several other successful experiments at the Pittsburgh facility furnish additional possibilities for hospital administrators concerned with helath planning. The Pittsburgh facility, for example, places personnel in local community hospitals to help upgrade their capacity to provide secondary care. In this way the Pittsburgh hospital recruited and paid a radiation physicist to work in a suburban institution, an addition that enhances the peripheral hospital's ability to provide area residents with radiation therapy. Similarly, the Pittsburgh facility has placed managerial personnel in the region's peripheral institutions to help solve fiscal and other administrative problems. Concrete steps like these, which assist the ability of the community hospital to provide secondary care, also encourage attending physicians to refer cases requiring tertiary care to the university-affiliated center. According to a representative of the Pittsburgh facility, outreach programs including concrete elements of this kind are more effective than efforts encompassing only educational initiatives. First, they promote in-house support at the community hospitals for referral of patients to the central facility. Second, they help create institution-to-institution rather than person-to-person linkages. "Linkages between institutions are more reliable than linkages between individuals," a spokesman commented. "Individual doctors retire, die, and have a tendency to become alienated from each other. Institutions are much more stable than people."

### The Insurance Industry

The insurance industry has more to gain from successful programs directed against cancer and other modern diseases than perhaps any other institution in the health care system. Lower death and disability rates from cancer would immediately reduce the liabilities for firms underwriting health plans or selling life insurance. An institution as important to health care as insurance has many means at its disposal for influencing the manner by which health care providers deliver their services. Insurance companies, for example, could encourage the formation of particular types of group practice among physicians by offering members of such groups favorable rates on malpractice policies. It is true that group practice is becoming an increasingly popular organizational form for American physicians. But little or no evidence exists in the health care literature that these group practices make it easier for cancer patients to receive the broad range of services they need within one group of physicians. Such an advantage would be offered only by groups of physicians including practitioners in several specialities. A specifically cancer-oriented group practice, for example, might include an oncologist, a surgeon, and a radiation therapist. Such an arrangement would facilitate the exchange of information among practitioners responsible for the same patient at different stages of the illness and coordinate their activities. A group practice consisting of only internists would be less effective in this sense, requiring that patients be referred outside the group whenever they needed surgery or radiation therapy. An informed insurance industry, therefore, would target its efforts on only the specific forms of group practice determined to effectively represent the social technology needed for control of cancer and other modern diseases. The insurance industry could, of course, offer lower premiums to individuals who underwent cancer screening or made visits to physicians for preventive purposes. Perhaps the insurance industry has already taken steps in this direction.

### Health Care Professionals

Physicians can contribute to cancer control in obvious ways, such as maintaining knowledge of current developments in cancer detection and treatment and improving their sensitivity to the need for patient referral. Less obviously, they could improve their ability to make the cancer patient more comfortable with the illness by facing the issue of death more directly and letting the patient know the likely course of the illness and the consequences of planned therapy for the patient's style of life. But the physician's most important contribution to cancer control beyond his or her individual area of responsibility might be in relations with nurses and other nonphysician health personnel. If the doctor provides supportive colleague relationships to the nurse attempting to provide emotional support for cancer patients, the nurse's ability to perform this difficult yet crucial function will increase. If the physician discourages such activity or even provides mere passive support, only the strongest, most committed nurses will be able to aid the patient's emotional adjustment, others either avoiding such tasks or seeking positions inside or outside nursing that are less demanding. As Chapter 6 suggests, emotional support is most effective when combined with intimate physical care for the patient. Since nurses already provide such physical care, they are the natural candidates for the emotional support role. Only the physician's encouragement can permit them to play the best role possible in emotional support.

Nurses themselves may advance the goals of cancer control in a seemingly self-serving way. By increasing their power relative to physicians, they will feel freer to perform the emotional adjustment role. By building a more prestigious profession through the usual political mechanisms of independent licensure, they may create more interesting and financially rewarding jobs in nursing careers. If such developments would reduce turnover on nursing staffs, individuals with advanced skills and experience would remain in bedside nursing far more often than they appear to at present.

The physician, however, still stands at the pivot of the health care system and affects the ability of programs like cancer control to succeed more than any other professional. Even without an explicit planning role, the physician at a regional medical center affects the outcome of regional planning efforts by his or her day-to-day activity. In a field bound by tradition and as conscious of status as medicine, there is no substitute for conscientious cultivation of trust and goodwill among community physicians. Again, this activity may take the form of simply keeping community physicians informed of the treatment their patients receive at the regional center. But even an activity this straightforward seems to require a degree of finesse. Commenting on his department's successes in attracting referrals, a radiotherapist at the university medical center explained:

> It is necessary to send each physician who refers a patient here a *personal letter* back. They don't respond well to forms, printouts, or anything standardized like that. They also don't like little mistakes like having their names spelled wrong or errors in their zip codes. The communication process takes a lot of time, and must be done by the specific department to which the patient is referred.

Curiously, this physician did not seem to know that the university medical center maintained a specialized liaison office for contacting referring physicians, but took the task of communication upon himself.

Successful planning efforts often seem to depend on careful cultivation of this nature. A university rheumatology clinic on the West Coast, for example, owes much of its success to the personal efforts of its director to cultivate durable relationships with his colleagues in the community. These efforts take the form of attending local medical society meetings as well as keeping in close communication when patients are actually referred. An effort to achieve better co-ordination of services at a university-affiliated health maintenance organization on the East Coast took a similar form. University personnel spent much time in close contact with practitioners, convincing them of the program's value and calming their fears that an associated reporting system would interfere with their independence.

Limited as they seem, these actions by individuals or individual institutions can initiate successful efforts toward cancer control. Means are available for use by creative planners in a variety of roles. Unfortunately, progress initiated by even creative and conscientious individuals will always face serious limitations by prevailing patterns of power and resource allocation that fit the needs of a society threatened by infectious ailments better than one primarily concerned with modern disease.

## LINGERING DOUBTS

Finally, it seems essential to examine the basic assumptions that underlie policy recommendations made here and in similar studies. The major planning issues with which this chapter began focused on structural considerations, that is, the more durable, concrete patterns of social relationships that govern the nation's health care system as a whole. Altering at least some of these relationships is clearly necessary for improved health care in cancer or any other disease. To emphasize major problems in creating a social technology capable of translating "state of the art" medical techniques into actual patient care and recommend concrete strategies, the preceding discussion temporarily accepted several familiar suppositions without question. No discussion of this kind would be complete, however, without examining these presuppositions, for they affect the validity of the recommended policy options and involve fundamental issues of social values.

First, it is necessary to hold the assumptions of Alford and Bodenheimer problematical. The preceding discussion fundamentally accepts their position, that is, existing patterns of power and resource allocation constitute the most important sources of frustration for those who introduce innovations into health care in the United States. But the exclusive focus that these two observers place on institutions peculiar to the United States does not tell the whole story. While important, the private practice-based, pluralistically organized features of health care in the contemporary United States do not account fully for the system's inability to provide coordinated services and continuity of care for victims of cancer and other modern diseases. Societies utilizing very different systems for the delivery of health care encounter at least some of the same problems.

Health care in the Soviet Union provides perhaps the best illustration. At least on paper, the Soviet health care system is structured in a manner that should avoid many of the difficulties this study has identified in cancer control. In the Soviet Union, for example, most health services are provided by physicians working in multiple purpose clinics attached to district hospitals.[12] Outpatient units are typically located within hospital buildings and administered as part of the hospital even when they are physically located outside it.[13] The implication that geographical and administrative integration should promote continuity of patient care is reinforced by the decided lack of pluralism in Soviet medicine. As Freidson writes:

> Physicians hold positions created and sustained by the state, with . . . little opportunity for private practice. Furthermore, their positions are salaried; the salaries are set by decree. Their working hours are determined bureaucratically (generally at 6½ hours per day), and bureaucratic norms are established to set the tempo of their work (in 1960, for example, pediatricians were expected to see an *average* of five patients per outpatient clinic hour). What is perhaps most important . . . however, is that the physician may appear to be almost wholly a creature of the state in that he has almost no sociopolitically independent position from which to stand outside the state.[14]

Reports on the functioning of the Soviet health care system, though, suggest that it shares some of the most important difficulties encountered by American medicine in its attempt to control modern disease. While urban dwellers in the Soviet Union appear to enjoy better access to primary care than those in Central City's District 11, provision of specialized services appears imperfectly coordinated with community practice in both localities. Ryan notes that all urban dwellers in the Soviet Union receive primary care from "sector physicians." But he observes that individuals referred to specialists may not be regarded by the specialists as patients of the sector doctor and that the sector doctor may not be kept fully informed about them. A quotation selected by Ryan from a Soviet medical journal is reminiscent of some of the major difficulties identified by the District 11 study facing health planners in Central City:

It is no secret that unwise use of the principle of specialization frequently results in the patient traipsing from one specialist to another, each one of whom prescribes different courses of treatment, some of which conflict.[15]

Fragmentation of this kind is only one consequence traceable to imperfections in regionalization efforts. But, as Chapter 2 notes in detail, this difficulty is especially important for successful control of cancer and other modern diseases on a regionwide basis. Contrary to the thinking of Alford and Bodenheimer, the problem of fragmentation does not appear to result entirely from the desire of physicians to reap ever-greater private incomes and hospitals to protect their independence. If Soviet doctors earn any income from private practice, it is probably minor; Soviet hospitals, under the direction of the Ministry of Health, have little independence to protect. A factor that helps explain fragmentation in both the United States and the Soviet Union may be the intellectual presuppositions that underlie specialization, allowing specialists to place low priority upon keeping primary care physicians or practitioners in other specialities informed about their activity. As Freidson concludes in a comparison of medicine in the United States, Britain, and the Soviet Union, medical expertise in all three societies "seems to have its own leverage."[16] An important implication for planners concerned with modern disease in the United States is that ideologies and status claims of specialists must be considered along with more concrete structural considerations in the formulation of programs for regional coordination.

Second, planners must question the nearly universal assumption that the university medical center should serve as the central focus and guiding influence in regional cancer control programs. If the Central City University facility is typical of university medical centers, a reconsideration may be in order. As Chapter 4 reports, this organization has a particularly strong ability to attract patients with specific types of cancer from distant locations, but it exerts no special drawing power upon individuals with the types of cancer that occur most frequently in its immediate locale. Leukemia and lymphomas, for example, account for a relatively small proportion (about 8 percent) of cancer cases nationwide.[17] Among cancer patients seen at the Central City University Medical Center in 1976 who resided in its immediate vicinity (District 11), only a minor proportion (less than 2 percent) suffered from leukemia and lymphoma. Yet among cancer patients residing outside Central City and vicinity, leukemia and lymphoma sufferers constituted more substantial percentages. Of the cases originating outside the Central City region, leukemia patients constituted 9.4 percent, Hodgkin's disease patients

4.7 percent, and non-Hodgkin's lymphomas patients 10.7 percent. In contrast, the medical center is no more likely to draw breast cancer cases from its immediate locale than from outside the Central City region. While breast cancer cases constituted 11.7 percent ($N = 22$) of the cancer patients residing in District 11, 13.4 percent ($N = 20$) of the cancer patients coming from outside the region had breast malignancies.

The mixture of cancer cases seen at the university medical center is an indication of its special capacities for treating different forms of the disease. Apparently, patients and their physicians at distant sites recognize the special ability of the medical center to treat leukemia and lymphoma. Physicians are willing to make referrals and patients to make long journeys to receive this specialized care. On the other hand, patients living in District 11 seem to make no special effort to receive treatment at the university medical center for breast cancer. The percentage of cancer patients seen at the center with malignancies of the breast is about equal to the percentage of cancer cases they represent nationwide. Assuming that physicians and patients perceive the offerings of the university medical center accurately, no special capacity appears available for treating the more common cancers, such as breast, prostate, and uterus. But outstanding therapy does seem to be available for other malignancies occurring less frequently in the population, such as leukemia and lymphoma.

Given these considerations, it may be more accurate to characterize the university facility as a *sectional* rather than a regional center. Within its immediate region, cancer patients may in fact receive service at many other sites for the most common cancers that is as effective as what the university has to offer. But patients from all over the Midwest seek care at the university for other, less common diseases. The unique contribution of the university medical center, then, seems to be in serving sectional rather than regional needs.

These considerations suggest that Central City University should not be the focal point for regional cancer control in the surrounding region. The social relations among physicians that facilitate referrals from the immediate locale take a different form from those connecting university physicians with practitioners at distant locations. Central City University clearly deserves considerable support from federal funding agencies, not only for its bench research, but also for cancer control on a sectional level. But it seems likely that an institution with a base more clearly regional in character would maintain the close ties with community physicians necessary for regional coordination more frequently than the Central City University.

Third, it seems important to examine the assumption made here and elsewhere that a greater sharing of responsibilities among health professionals would be beneficial to victims of cancer and other modern diseases. As suggested earlier, the sense of personal responsibility that plays so important a part in the physician's training has several clear functions. The physician, of course, must take decisive action in emergency situations. But the sense of personal responsibility by the physician is important for less technical reasons as well. As Chapter 6 notes, the most conscientious physician plays the part of "anchor man" on the health care team, accepting final responsibility for all the care that the cancer patient receives, answering the patient's questions about his or her condition, and providing valuable elements of emotional support. Analysts must ask whether a weakened sense of final responsibility for the patient by a single physician would not make this role more difficult to assume. Anything less than full, final responsibility for the crucial features of cancer management may be insufficient to motivate physicians to perform the challenging functions of coordination and emotional support that many physicians now accept.

Two policy recommendations implied and specified throughout this volume bear on the physician's sense of final responsibility in cancer management. First, the notion that treatment of modern disease requires more than one doctor contradicts the important medical tradition of individual responsibility. Second, the recommendation that nurses assume greater initiative and discretion in patient care may create a sense of rivalry between physician and nurse. This could become especially serious if, as suggested earlier in this chapter, nurses adopted an aggressive strategy aimed at upgrading their positions as professionals. Such a strategy may induce otherwise highly committed physicians to withdraw from the central position they now occupy in the less technical aspects of cancer management.

From the policymaker's point of view, the best alternative would be a replacement of the professional dominance of physicians by more cooperative relations between nurses and doctors. As Strauss and others suggest, this cooperative relationship often exists already under the rapidly changing conditions that prevail on wards for the treatment of seriously ill patients. As a social objective, this sense of cooperation must become reliable and general. Whether this goal is in fact achieved will depend largely on the approach that nurses and physicians adopt to alterations in the power relationships between them. An overly militant stance among nurses will induce at least some physicians to withdraw from useful functions they now perform, whereas a rigid response from physicians will help perpetuate the problem of turnover among highly qualified nursing personnel.

Perhaps the most problematical assumptions made in this study concern the traditional relations among patients, physicians, and families. On the basis of the Professional Community Survey, Chapter 6 questions the efficacy of traditional sources of emotional support, the patient's family and physician. Efforts by policymakers to act on these conclusions call into question some of the most highly prized institutions of American society and oldest values of humankind. A cancer control program that allocated resources for improvement of the emotional dimension of care for cancer patients without taking the importance of these traditions into consideration would be misdirected. Recognition of these traditional roles is hardly incompatible with solutions to the problems created by modern disease. Other modern societies, particularly Japan, have recognized the ability of family members to provide unique forms of support to their dying kinsmen; hospitals in Japan make special provisions to allow family members to provide intimate physical care for terminal patients.[18] It is highly problematical whether public policy should encourage the replacement of grieving kin with sympathetic professionals armed with hypodermic needles. Yet a cancer control program that trained professionals but not families to care for the dying might do exactly that.

The best strategies for cancer control programs may seek a compromise between the needs associated with modern disease and the benefits available from traditional relationships and institutions. Some approaches to the emotional needs of modern disease victims are clearly undesirable from this perspective. Several writers, for example, have urged the establishment of a group of professionals called "intervention workers" in terminal cancer units for the purpose of meeting both the patient's and family's emotional needs.[19] Analysts must wonder, though, whether creating a new class of professionals is appropriate. Families may consider such personnel superfluous, gravitating toward physicians and nurses whose traditional functions they comprehend and value. As suggested above, upgrading the nurse may be the best strategy because the professional values of nursing are highly compatible with emotional support. In addition, proposals to aid the patient and family through mutual peer support[20] seem highly attractive, strengthening traditional social relationships and preserving individual autonomy through knowledgeable professional assistance. Still, planners and policymakers must remember that many cancer patients will depend fully on health care professionals for emotional support. As the number of homebound elderly citizens in modern American society indicates, demographic factors make the physical presence of concerned family members at the cancer patient's bedside far from universal.[21]

Finally, and perhaps fundamentally, policy analysts must ask how clearly cancer control efforts can be separated from other functions of the health care system. Like many other federal programs, cancer control is essentially categorical in nature, focusing on a specific problem area rather than attempting to deal with several interrelated problems at once. This degree of categorization often entails serious dysfunctions in other social programs. Public employment programs, for example, typically overlook health problems that prevent people from taking jobs. A similar difficulty may apply in cancer control. Although legislators have earmarked funds for this specific category of disease, its large-scale management may be impossible or at least considerably more difficult if not integrated into the more general functions of the health care system. Perhaps the best illustration of dysfunctions that may arise from "overcategorization" is apparent in cancer screening. Chapter 7 strongly suggests that lack of integration of cancer screening facilities into the wider health care system discourages patients with suspicious symptoms from following up their visits to screening centers with visits to physicians. A more serious problem may occur among individuals who do not seek screening for specific illnesses in the absence of visible symptoms. Two prominent observers suggest that the best method for providing these individuals with screening services is to include them in the course of regular medical examinations. But these observers also recognize that many persons in high-risk categories are infrequent users of routine medical services.[22] Clearly, effective cancer control cannot be confined in focus to malignancies alone if it is to benefit these segments of the population.

## NOTES

1. T.S. Bodenheimer, "Regional Medical Programs: No Road to Regionalization," *Medical Care Review* 26 (1969): 1125–1166. See p. 1131.

2. Ibid., p. 1130.

3. Ibid., p. 1142.

4. Ibid.

5. Robert R. Alford, Health Care Politics (Chicago: University of Chicago Press, 1975), p. 14.

6. Bodenheimer, op. cit., p. 1143.

7. Ibid., p. 1144.

8. A.L. Strauss, "Structure and Ideology of the Nursing Profession," in Fred Davis, (ed.), *The Nursing Profession* (New York: John Wiley, 1966), pp. 60-104.

9. Ibid., p. 84.

10. Anselm L. Strauss and Barney G. Glaser, *Time for Dying* (Chicago: Aldine Publishing Co., 1968).

11. A. Wildavsky, "Can Health Care Be Planned?" (Michael M. Davis Lecture, Chicago: Center for Health Administration Studies, 1976).

12. Eliot Freidson, *Profession of Medicine* (New York: Dodd, Mead and Co., 1975), p. 41.

13. Michael Ryan, *The Organization of Soviet Medical Care* (Oxford: Basil Blackwell and London: Martin Robertson, 1978), p. 79.

14. Freidson, op. cit., p. 41.

15. Ryan, op. cit., p. 90.

16. Freidson, op. cit., p. 43.

17. American Cancer Society, *1977 Cancer Facts and Figures* (Chicago: American Cancer Society, 1976), p. 9.

18. Strauss and Glaser, op. cit.

19. M.J. Krant et al. "The Role of a Hospital-Based Psychosocial Unit in Terminal Cancer Illness and Bereavement," *Journal of Chronic Disease* 29 (1976): 115-127.

20. See, for example, M.A. Lieberman and G.R. Bond, "Self-Help Groups," *Small Group Behavior* 9 (May 1978): 221-241; M.P. DuMont, "Self-Help Treatment Programs," *American Journal of Psychiatry* 6 (June 1974): 631-635.

21. Philip W. Buchner, *Home Health Care for the Aged* (New York: Appleton-Century-Crofts, 1978), pp. 3-7.

22. R.B. Warnecke, and S. Graham, "Characteristics of Blacks Obtaining Papanicolaou Smears," *Cancer* 37 (1976): 2015-2025.

# Appendix: Research Methods and Instruments

In general, the research methods that generated data for the study reported above follow the tradition of the "unique case study." No region in the United States is likely to duplicate the Central City Cancer Control Program service region in exact detail; while the Metropolitan Screening Clinic resembles other early detection facilities in various parts of the United States, subtle yet important features may distinguish it from its counterparts. Strictly speaking, the data collected on professionals at the Central City University Medical Center and the eleven hospitals associated with it for cancer control represent only professionals at these twelve institutions; similarly, the clients of the Metropolitan Screening Clinic interviewed in this study represent only those who exhibited symptoms possibly indicating cancer, yet whose cases remained closed in the clinic records. While the resulting data may not be generalized directly to other universes of professionals or patients, they are entirely adequate for the purposes of this volume. Again, the aim of this book is to develop strong hypotheses about the social factors that limit the success of cancer control and related programs as initiated in federal legislation and provide suggestions for planners interested in overcoming these barriers. The unique case study is classically recognized as an appropriate method for generating ideas of this kind,[1] and many outstanding sociological investigations have utilized the form.[2] Although they do not necessarily reflect conditions outside the cancer control program service region, the data presented here should provide useful insights to planners of regional health services everywhere.

The Professional Community Survey furnished the greatest volume of numerical data for this book. This component of the research provided an understanding of the opinions and perceptions of "cancer-oriented staff" at the university medical center and eleven associated community hospitals. The survey proceeded in a "snowball" fashion, commencing with interviews at each hospital of heads of the departments of medicine, surgery, pediatrics, radiology, and nursing. After interviewing these individuals, researchers requested them to recommend colleagues in their departments with special interests in cancer care. The survey generally included at least two individuals in each of the areas specified, although larger numbers of individuals in each category were interviewed at the university medical center. Physicians, nurses, chaplains, and social workers were selected in this way and requested to answer questions about goals, attitudes, collegial relationships, and, in the case of doctors, types of cancer most frequently encountered. Finally, researchers interviewed the head of medical records, the chief hospital administrator, the chief pathologist, and the chief pharmacist at each hospital in order to collect data on available medications and resources. With the inclusion of 50 radiology outpatients, total respondents numbered 414. As readers have undoubtedly noticed by this time, only the data on physicians and nurses have been presented in this volume. The other categories of respondents have been omitted, not because they are unimportant, but to simplify the task of data analysis while retaining a perspective on the difference between physicians and nonphysicians. The schedule of questions used in the Professional Community Survey appears below.

All interviewing in the Professional Community Survey took place on a face-to-face basis with interviewers actively involved in assisting subjects to answer questions on the interview schedule. Many physicians encountered questions that they did not think applied well to their practice and declined to answer these items. This necessitated careful separation of indications of nonapplicability from negative answers in the data analysis. Some physicians resisted the research effort, a few taking the time to read the questions but expressing critical comments about the survey and its sponsors instead of providing answers. These individuals, though, were few in number and separable in the data analysis from those who provided valid answers to items in the interview.

The Professional Community Survey aimed at determining the characteristics, practices, and attitudes of a very specific population of health care workers—those whose organizations expressed a willingness to cooperate in the university's efforts to establish a regional system for promoting cancer control. The hospitals surveyed, once again, represent neither a random sample of local hospitals, nor a population of hospitals whose characteristics are strictly generalizable to any other specific set of similar organizations. Rather, they constitute a population of hospitals with at least some staff members actively interested in promoting regional cancer control through participation in a university-led and educationally based effort, and whose professional and administrative leadership was willing to commit staff time to associated activities. These hospitals are distinctly different from others in the area that either refused to participate in the survey or never received requests to participate. Generally, they had some preexisting ties to the university in the form of professional relations with cancer specialists there. Most participated or planned at some point to participate in the university's educational outreach program for community physicians. These features of the hospitals surveyed suggest that they have stronger commitments to cancer detection and treatment and improving these functions through continuing professional education than most hospitals in the area.

The sampling approach used here is especially valuable in research related to policy questions in cancer control. Because the individuals surveyed were drawn from organizations particularly favorable to innovation in cancer-related activites, problems visible among them would be quite likely to occur among professionals in work groups less favorable to change. Because the innovation proposed involves minimum fiscal or administrative impact upon the professionals and organizations at which it aims, programs making more concrete demands on health care personnel and hospitals would almost certainly encounter at least as much resistance. The study described in this book provides scholars and policymakers with a reliable indication of the difficulties they would be most likely to expect in implementing even the most limited regional health care plan under the most favorable conceivable conditions.

Although the cancer control project represented a creative and innovative approach to regional health planning and received enthusiastic support in some quarters of the community, this book emphasizes problems that could have limited its success had the program continued beyond its closing date. In this sense, readers should view the research reported here as an evaluation of a "prospective" nature. Because the cancer control program was essentially a demonstration project of short duration, no "before-after" data could be collected to systematically test the outcome of the program. Instead, the research effort focused on the structure and process of medical care related to cancer in the cooperating hospitals, an approach of widely recognized utility in the absence of outcome data.

The investigation of clients at the Metropolitan Screening Clinic utilized two approaches, structured interviews performed over the telephone of 300 clients of the clinic and thirty in-depth interviews performed with clients on a face-to-face basis. Because these methods have received detailed attention in Chapter 7, they will not be further considered here. The questionnaire used in the telephone interviewing and the schedule of items used in the face-to-face procedure, however, appear below.

# PROFESSIONAL COMMUNITY SURVEY

1.0 GOALS

All of the following goals regarding cancer are important. However, some are stressed more than others, depending on the institution, its resources, and the people it serves.

In your opinion, please rate each of the following goals according to its importance in your institution. That is, the more important the goal, the more effort, time, and money will be spent to achieve it.

RATING (1,2,3,4, according to key below)*

| | | |
|---|---|---|
| 1.1 | Identify people at risk (i.e., for cancer of skin, lung, cervix) | _____ |
| 1.2 | Early Detection and Screening of cancer | _____ |
| 1.3 | Diagnosis of Cancer | _____ |
| 1.4 | Treatment of Cancer | _____ |
| 1.5 | Continuing patient care (other than primary diagnosis and treatment) | _____ |
| | Referral to appropriate patient care: | |
| 1.6 | ...within institution | _____ |
| 1.7 | ...outside institution | _____ |
| 1.8 | Physical Rehabilitation of cancer patients | _____ |
| 1.9 | Social-Psychological help to cancer patients and/or their families | _____ |
| 1.10 | Encourage regular and scheduled screening | _____ |
| 1.11 | Cancer education for in-hospital patients | _____ |
| 1.12 | Cancer education for health professionals | _____ |
| 1.13 | Cancer research | _____ |
| 1.14 | Fund raising for cancer research and education | _____ |

* 1. Very much effort, time, and money is spent to achieve this goal
  2. A fair amount of effort, time and money is spent to achieve this goal.
  3. Some effort, time, and money is spent to achieve this goal.
  4. Hardly any effort, time and money is spent to achieve this goal.

A-8

## 2.0 PREVENTION

2.1 Are any cancer prevention programs offered by this institution? _____
If no, go on to 3.0

2.2     For which cancer sites are prevention programs available:

.1 _____

.2 _____

.3 _____

2.3     Please describe the program (s):

_____

_____

Whom is this program aimed at (i.e. industrial workers,
elderly, students, women, smokers,etc.)

Approximate # of people reached:

2.4.1 _____     2.4.2 _____

2.5.1 _____     2.5.2 _____

2.6.1 _____     2.6.2 _____

2.7 Please feel free to discuss any problems (and possible solutions) you have
encountered in setting up and running your cancer prevention program(s).

_____

_____

_____

A-9

### 3.0 SCREENING

3.1.1  Is there a fully integrated cancer screening clinic run by this institution? _____

3.1.2  Are any cancer screening programs offered by this institution?_____

(If no to both, go on to 4.0)

Please describe screening program(s):

| .1<br>Cancer Sites | .2<br>Target Pop. | .3<br>Approximate number of people<br>screened in last year |
|---|---|---|
| 3.2 _____ | _____ | _____ |
| 3.3 _____ | _____ | _____ |
| 3.4 _____ | _____ | _____ |

3.5  How often are the screening programs offered? _____

3.6  Are there any provisions for follow-up? _____

(If no, go on to 3.9)

3.7.1  Is follow-up carried on in your institution? _____

3.7.2  Is follow-up carried on by referral? _____

(If no, go on to 3.9)

3.8  If referral is used for follow-up, to whom or where are referrals usually made?

_____

_____

3.9  What types of publicity are employed for the screening programs? (Check those used)

.1  Paid newspaper advertisements _____

.2  P-R releases to newspapers _____

.3  Radio _____

.4  Television _____

.5  In-hospital fliers _____

.6  Community fliers _____

.7  Other (_____) _____

3.10  Please circle the type of publicity which you have found most effective

Who staffs your screening programs:

Number _____

3.11  Physicians _____

3.12  Nurses _____

3.13  Other staff - i.e. Secretaries
                      Technicians _____

3.14  Volunteers _____

3.15  Please feel free to discuss any problems (and possible solutions) you have encountered in setting up and running your screening program.

_____

_____

A-10

## 4.0 REHABILITATION

4.1 Are any rehabilitation services offered by this institution? _____
(If no, go on to 5.0.)

For what cancer sites is rehabilitation available:

|  | .1<br>Cancer Sites | .2<br>Approximate number of<br>people using service<br>in past year |
|---|---|---|
| 4.2 | _____ | _____ |
| 4.3 | _____ | _____ |
| 4.4 | _____ | _____ |

4.5 At what stage in the cancer patient's treatment is patient first made aware of this service? (check one)

      pre-hospital admission    _____

      pre-op in hospital    _____

      post-op in hospital    _____

      post-hospital discharge    _____

4.6 By whom is referral of patient to rehabilitation service usually made? (check one)

| M.D. | _____ | Chaplain | _____ |
|---|---|---|---|
| Nurse | _____ | Self | _____ |
| Social Worker | _____ | Family | _____ |
| Other (_____) | _____ | | |

4.7 Who else may occasionally refer patient? (Circle appropriate in 4.6).

4.8 Is the rehabilitation program free of charge to patients? _____
If no, go on to No.4.10.

4.9 How is the rehabilitation program financed if free of charge to patient?
That is, how is the patient subsidized?

                                                   Check Source(s)

    .1 State funds    _____

    .2 National funds    _____

    .3 Other agency. Specify (_____) _____

4.10 Please feel free to discuss any problems (and possible solutions) you have encountered in setting up and running your rehabilitation program.

_____

_____

A-11

## 5.0 CONTINUING CARE

5.1 Are there any continuing care programs offered by this institution to the cancer patient <u>in the</u> home? _____
(If no, go on to 5.17)

5.2 Does this care include the patient's family? _____
If no, go on to 5.3).
If yes, explain briefly how the family is included.

_____

_____

5.3 What types of continuing care are offered?

|  |  | Check if offered |
|---|---|---|
| .1 | homemaker service | _____ |
| .2 | public health nurse visits | _____ |
| .3 | social worker visits | _____ |
| .4 | agency or hospital-based support groups for patient | _____ |
| .5 | other support groups for patient | _____ |
| .6 | agency or hospital-based support groups for patient's family | _____ |
| .7 | agency or hospital-based groups for patient's family | _____ |
| .8 | other (_____) | _____ |

5.4 By whom is referral of patient (and/or family) <u>usually</u> made? (check one)

| Physician | _____ | Agency or Hospital Discharge Planner | _____ |
|---|---|---|---|
| Hospital nurse | _____ | | |
| Public Health Nurse | _____ | American Cancer Society Representative | _____ |
| Medical Social Worker | _____ | Other patients | _____ |
| Other (_____) | _____ | Patient Self referral | _____ |

5.5 Who else may occasionally refer patient (Circle appropriate in 5.4)

5.6 Do you charge the patient for the continuing care service? _____
(If no, go on to 5.9).

5.7 How do patients usually finance these services? (check if appropriate)

| .1 | Savings and personal loans | _____ |
|---|---|---|
| .2 | Medical insurance | _____ |
| .3 | Public Aid (Medicare/Medicard) | _____ |
| .4 | Other (_____) | _____ |

A-12

9.0   SELECTED CANCERS

Please estimate the frequency with which you have diagnosed
the following in the past year. (leave blank those that are not relevant to your practice).
(For interviewer: Ask by topic first; if none seen go on to next group)

| | | .1 Number Diagnosed | | If you usually did not manage all stages of this cancer, where did you usually refer case? |
| | 1-3 | 4-10 | 11+ | |
|---|---|---|---|---|
| **SKIN** | | | | |
| 9.1   squamous cell carcinoma | | | | |
| 9.2   basal cell carcinoma | | | | |
| 9.3   melanoma | | | | |
| **HEAD AND NECK** | | | | |
| 9.4   mouth and floor of mouth | | | | |
| 9.5   tongue | | | | |
| 9.6   tonsil | | | | |
| 9.7   larynx | | | | |
| 9.8   nasopharynx | | | | |
| 9.9   sinuses | | | | |
| 9.10  parotid | | | | |
| 9.11  hypopharynx | | | | |
| 9.12  hard and soft palate | | | | |
| 9.13  other salivary gland tumors | | | | |
| **THORAX** | | | | |
| 9.14  esophagus | | | | |
| 9.15  lung | | | | |
| **BREAST** | | | | |
| 9.16  breast | | | | |
| **GASTROINTESTINAL** | | | | |
| 9.17  pancreas (including insulinomas/Zollinger-Ellison tumors | | | | |
| 9.18  liver | | | | |
| 9.19  gall bladder | | | | |
| 9.20  stomach | | | | |
| 9.21  small bowel | | | | |
| 9.22  colon | | | | |
| 9.23  Rectum and anus | | | | |

A-13

9.0 - SELECTED CANCERS (continued)

| | .1 Number Diagnosed | | | .2 If you usually did not manage all stages of this cancer, where did you usually refer case? |
|---|---|---|---|---|
| | 1-3 | 4-10 | 11+ | |
| ENDOCRINE | | | | |
| 9.24  thyroid | | | | |
| 9.25  parathyroid | | | | |
| 9.26  adrenal | | | | |
| UROLOGY | | | | |
| 9.27  kidney | | | | |
| 9.28  prostate | | | | |
| 9.29  bladder | | | | |
| 9.30  testicles | | | | |
| 9.31  penis | | | | |
| GYNECOLOGY | | | | |
| 9.32  uterus -cervix and corpus | | | | |
| 9.33  tube | | | | |
| 9.34  ovary | | | | |
| 9.35  vulva | | | | |
| 9.36  vagina | | | | |
| CNS | | | | |
| 9.37  brain | | | | |
| 9.38  spinal cord | | | | |
| LYMPHOMAS | | | | |
| 9.39  Hodgkin's | | | | |
| 9.40  non-Hodgkin's lymphomas | | | | |
| HEMATOLOGICAL MALIGNANCIES | | | | |
| 9.41  leukemia - chronic | | | | |
| 9.42  leukemia - acute | | | | |
| 9.43  plasma cell neoplasm | | | | |

A-14

## 9.0 - SELECTED CANCERS (continued)

| | | .1 Number Diagnoses | | | .2 If you usually did not manage all stages of this cancer, where did you usually refer case? |
| --- | --- | --- | --- | --- | --- |
| | | 1-3 | 4-10 | 11+ | |
| **CHILDHOOD TUMORS** | | | | | |
| 9.44 | acute childhood leukemia | | | | |
| 9.45 | brain tumor | | | | |
| 9.46 | Hodgkin's disease and lymphoma | | | | |
| 9.47 | non-Hodgkin's lymphoma | | | | |
| 9.48 | neuroblastoma | | | | |
| 9.49 | Wilm's tumor | | | | |
| 9.50 | bone cancer | | | | |
| 9.51 | liver cancer | | | | |
| 9.52 | retinoblastoma | | | | |
| 9.53 | rhabomyosarcoma | | | | |

A-15

11.0  METASTATIC PROBLEMS

What percent of the cancer patients you see?

11.1  have metastatic problems  at first contact: _____ %

11.2  develop metastatic problems? _____ %

Approximately how many patients with metastatic problems have you seen in the past year:

11.3  Approximate number treated in past year  _____

11.4  Approximate number referred in past year  _____

Please check the usual methods you use when treating metastatic problems

| FOR: | .1  SURGERY | .2 RADIOTHERAPY | .3 CHEMOTHERAPY | .4 STEROIDS |
|---|---|---|---|---|
| 11.5 Spinal cord compression | | | | |
| 11.6 Brain metastasis | | | | |
| 11.7 Malignant effusions | | | | |

11.8  If you sometimes refer patients with metastatic problems, where do you usually refer them?

.1 _____

.2 _____

A-16

Approximate number of patients treated in the last year for:
13.1   palliative purposes _____
13.2   cure

_____

13.3   Is a radium stock available? _____

13.4   Are intracavity radium treatments performed? _____

13.5   Is a treatment simulator used in treatment planning? _____

How is dosimetry performed?

13.6     with a computer? _____      13.8   by outside consultation? _____

13.7     with a hand calculator? _____     (specify) _____

Are port films used in

13.9     planning? _____

13.10    treatment verification ? _____

Please check these pieces of equipment this hospital has and specify the year acquired.

|  |  | .1 Check if available here | .2 Year Acquired |
|---|---|---|---|
| 13.11 | Linear accelerator | _____ | _____ |
| 13.12 | Cobalt generator | _____ | _____ |
| 13.13 | Betatron | _____ | _____ |
| 13.14 | Van de Graaff generator | _____ | _____ |
| 13.15 | Orthovoltage machine | _____ | _____ |

13.16   Are radiotherapy facilities in any other hospital used? _____
   .   If yes, please specify:

      .1 Facility          and      .2 Location

13.17   _____      _____

13.18   _____      _____

A-17

## 16.0 SOCIAL SERVICE

16.1 Does this hospital receive any funds to aid in patient transportation from home to hospital? _____. (If no, go on to 16.4)

16.2 If yes, where are funds from?

.1 _____

.2 _____

16.3 If yes, how are funds used?

.1 _____

.2 _____

How does the cancer patient usually get to the hospital, especially when frequent visits are necessary?

| | Very Often | Fairly Often | Occasion- ally | Hardly Ever | Nev |
|---|---|---|---|---|---|
| 16.4    Patients arrange own transportation | | | | | |
| 16.5    Hospital provides bus, cab, or limousine service | | | | | |
| 16.6    Hospital volunteers transport patients in own cars | | | | | |
| 16.7    Community or neighborhood groups (i.e. church members) volunteer to transport patients. | | | | | |
| 16.8    American Cancer Society provides transportation (i.e. cab service or volunteers). | | | | | |

16.9 Approximate number of cancer patients (and/or families) seen by social service in past month _____.

What is the nature of the social workers contact with cancer patients and/or their families?

| | Very Often | Fairly Often | Occasion- ally | Hardly Ever | Never |
|---|---|---|---|---|---|
| 16.10   discharge planning | | | | | |
| 16.11   arrange means of transportation | | | | | |
| 16.12   financial ability to pay bills | | | | | |
| 16.13   understand the nature of the disease | | | | | |
| 16.14   impact of disease on family and future | | | | | |
| 16.15   act as mediator or interpreter between doctor, nurse and patient, and patient's family. | | | | | |
| 16.16   other (_____) | | | | | |

A-18

## 25.0 COMMUNICATION

How often do you <u>discuss</u> cancer patient cases with the following:*

| | Very Often | Fairly Often | Occasionally | Hardly Ever | Never |
|---|---|---|---|---|---|
| Physicians: | | | | | |
| 25.1 oncologist - internist | | | | | |
| 25.2 surgeon | | | | | |
| 25.3 radiation therapist | | | | | |
| 25.4 other physician (specify) | | | | | |
| 25.5 Nurses | | | | | |
| 25.6 Other health workers (i.e., dietitian, therapist, etc.) | | | | | |
| 25.7 Hospital based Social Workers | | | | | |
| 25.8 Community based Social Workers | | | | | |
| 25.9 Community Agencies (i.e., VNA or A.C.S. "Reach for Recovery" | | | | | |
| 25.10 Chaplains | | | | | |
| 25.11 Family or friends of cancer patient | | | | | |
| 25.12 Other? | | | | | |

* Very often - 3 or more times a week
  Fairly often - 1 or 2 times a week
  Occasionally - 2 or 3 times a week
  Hardly ever - 1 time a month or less

23.0  CONSULTATION - INITIATED

How often do you ask the following persons or groups to see a specific person with cancer

|  | Very Often | Fairly Often | Occasionally | Hardly Ever | Never |
|---|---|---|---|---|---|
| Physicians: | | | | | |
| 23.1  oncologist - internist | | | | | |
| 23.2  surgeon | | | | | |
| 23.3  radiation therapist | | | | | |
| 23.4  other physician (specify) | | | | | |
| 23.5  Nurses | | | | | |
| 23.6  Other health workers (i.e., dietitian, therapist, etc.) | | | | | |
| 23.7  Hospital based Social Workers | | | | | |
| 23.8  Community based Social Workers | | | | | |
| 23.9  Community Agencies (i.e., VNA or A.C.S. "Reach for Recovery" | | | | | |
| 23.10  Chaplains | | | | | |
| 23.11  Family or friends of cancer patient | | | | | |
| 23.12  Other? | | | | | |

* Very often - 3 or more times a week
  Fairly often- 1 or 2 times a week
  Occasionally - 2 or 3 times a month
  Hardly ever - 1 time a month or less

A-20

## 24.0 CONSULTATION - RECIPIENT

How often are you asked by the following persons or groups to see a specific person with cancer _____.

| | Very Often | Fairly Often | Occasionally | Hardly Ever | Never |
|---|---|---|---|---|---|
| **Physicians:** | | | | | |
| 24.1 oncologist - internist | | | | | |
| 24.2 surgeon | | | | | |
| 24.3 radiation therapist | | | | | |
| 24.4 other physician (Specify) | | | | | |
| 24.5 Nurses | | | | | |
| 24.6 Other health workers (i.e., dietitian, therapist, etc.) | | | | | |
| 24.7 Hospital based Social Workers | | | | | |
| 24.8 Community based Social Workers | | | | | |
| 24.9 Community Agencies (i.e., VNA or A.C.S.) | | | | | |
| 24.10 Chaplains | | | | | |
| 24.11 Family or friends of cancer patient | | | | | |
| 24.12 The patient himself or herself "self-referral" | | | | | |
| 24.13 Other | | | | | |

*  Very often - 3 or more times a week
   Fairly often - 1 or 2 times a week
   Occasionally - 2 or 3 times a month
   Hardly ever - 1 time a month or less

<u>20.0  EDUCATION</u>

How many talks have you attended in the past year particularly concerning cancer? (If no talks were attended, go on to 20.13)

20.1  Number in this hospital_____          20.2  Topics:_____
                                                     _____

20.3  Number outside of this hospital_____   20.5  Topics:_____
20.4  Where?_____                       _____
      _____

20.6  Were you reimbursed financially for your attendance at these talks? _____
      If yes, please specify:

                                    .1 <u>Check, if yes</u>      .2  <u>By whom?</u>

      20.7  for registration fees   _____   _____

      20.8  for travel expenses     _____   _____

      20.9  for time off from work  _____   _____

20.10 Did you receive any formal recognition, advancement, or credit for attendance at these talks? _____

      If yes, please specify:  <u>.1 kind</u>      and      <u>.2  by whom</u>

              20.11  _____        _____

              20.12  _____        _____

20.13 What topics concerning cancer would you like to see covered in future programs or lectures?

              .1 _____

              .2 _____

              .3 _____

A-22

**22.0 PREPARATION**

My preparation in meeting the <u>physical</u> needs of the cancer patient has been:

(circle one)

22.1  <u>In professional school</u>          22.2  <u>Post-grad experience</u>

      excellent                                 excellent

      very good                                 very good

      good                                      good

      fair                                      fair

      poor                                      poor


My preparation in meeting the <u>emotional and psychological</u> needs of the cancer patient and his or her family has been:

22.3  <u>In professional school</u>          22.4  <u>Post-grad experience</u>

      excellent                                 excellent

      very good                                 very good

      good                                      good

      ·fair                                     fair

      poor                                      poor

_____

22.5  Year graduated from professional school _____

22.6  Number of years of post-grad experience as professional _____

A-23

### 27.0  ADJUSTMENT

Please put "1" next to the individual or group who you feel <u>should</u> play the most important part in helping the cancer patient emotionally adjust to his condition; "2" to the second most important part, etc.  (Rank 1 to 6 with "6" playing the least important part).

<u>Rank 1 through 6</u>

27.1  the patient's family                          _____

27.2  the chaplain and/or religious worker          _____

27.3  the nurse                                      _____

27.4  the doctor                                     _____

27.5  the social worker                              _____

27.6  someone else who has cancer                    _____

This next question is similar to the preceding one except now we would like to know, in your opinion, who <u>actually</u> does play the most important part in helping the cancer patient adjust, etc. in your own setting.

<u>Rank 1 through 6</u>

27.7  the patient's family                          _____

27.8  the chaplain and/or religious worker          _____

27.9  the nurse                                      _____

27.10  the doctor                                    _____

27.11 . the social worker                            _____

27.12  someone else who has cancer                   _____

A-24

## 28.0 ATTITUDES

28.1  Most of the people I care for who develop cancer:

   ...are prepared adequately to deal with it.

   | Strongly agree | Agree | Disagree | Strongly disagree |

28.2      ...are difficult to talk with about their condition

   | Strongly agree | Agree | Disagree | Strongly disagree |

23.3      ...should be told their diagnosis in clear, understandable terms as soon as possible.

   | Strongly agree | Agree | Disagree | Strongly disagree |

28.4      ...would prefer not to know too much about their condition, even though they say otherwise

   | Strongly agree | Agree | Disagree | Strongly disagree |

28.5      ...are more demanding of my time than other patients

   | Strongly agree | Agree | Disagree | Strongly disagree |

# METROPOLITAN SCREENING CLINIC STUDY

TELEPHONE INTERVIEW SCHEDULE

My name is _____. I'm calling on behalf
of the Metropolitan Screening Clinic.          As we said in
the letter we sent you last week, the clinic is trying to find ways to
improve its service. Could you help us by answering a few brief questions about your contact with the Clinic.

A.  First, we would like to know your reasons for visiting the clinic:

    1.a.  Were you required by your employer to visit the clinic?

        1. ☐ yes (ask 1.b.)   0. ☐ no (go to 2.a.)

    1.b.  Was this requirement very important, moderately important,
          slightly important, or not important at all in your decision
          to visit the clinic?

        1. ☐ Very important (skip to part B.)
        2. ☐ Moderately important ⎫ ask
        3. ☐ Slightly important ⎬ 2.a.
        4. ☐ Not important at all ⎭

    2.a.  Before you visited the clinic, did you have any symptoms
          such as pain, bleeding, a wart or a mole, which you thought
          might indicate serious illness?

        1. ☐ yes (ask 2.b.)   0. ☐ no (go to 3.a.)

    2.b.  Were these symptoms very important, moderately important,
          only slightly important, or not important at all in your
          decision to visit the clinic?

        1. ☐ Very important
        2. ☐ Moderately important
        3. ☐ Slightly important
        4. ☐ Not important at all

(4-7)

A-26

3.a. Did you visit the clinic as part of a periodic routine to maintain good health, which you would follow even if you had no symptoms of illness?

1. ☐ yes (ask 3.b.)     0.  ☐ no (go to 4.a.)

3.b. Was this periodic routine very important, moderately important, slightly important, or not important at all in your decision to visit the clinic?

1. ☐ Very important
2. ☐ Moderately important
3. ☐ Slightly important
4. ☐ Not important at all

4.a. Did a member of your family or someone else personally close to you help persuade you to visit the clinic?

1. ☐ yes (ask 4.b.)     0.  ☐ no (go to 5.a.)

4.b. Was this persuasion very important, moderately important, slightly important, or not important at all in your decision to visit the clinic?

1. ☐ Very important
2. ☐ Moderately important
3. ☐ Slightly important
4. ☐ Not important at all

5.a. Did a physician or other health care provider advise you to visit the clinic?

1. ☐ yes (ask 5.b.)     0.  ☐ no (go to 6)

5.b. Was this person a physician or another kind of health care provider?

1. ☐ Physician (ask question 5.c.)
2. ☐ Other health care provider
   SPECIFY _____

_____
_____ (skip to 5.d.)

A-27

5.c. Was this physician your regular family doctor or not?

1. ☐ Yes, regular family physician
2. ☐ No, other: SPECIFY _____
_____
_____

5.d. Was the (physician's or health care provider's) advice very important, moderately important, slightly important, or not important at all in your decision to visit the clinic?

1. ☐ Very important
2. ☐ Moderately important
3. ☐ Slightly important
4. ☐ Not important at all

6.a. Was your visit to the clinic paid for by an employer, insurance policy, or party other than yourself?

1. ☐ yes (ask 6.b. and c.)    0. ☐ no (go to part B.)

6.b. Who actually paid for your visit?

_____

_____

6.c. Was this payment arrangement very important, moderately important, slightly important, or not important at all in your decision to visit the clinic?

1. ☐ Very important
2. ☐ Moderately important
3. ☐ Slightly important
4. ☐ Not important at all

B. Next, we would like your opinion about some of the services the clinic offers.

1.a. First, on the day you visited the clinic, how much time do you recall being examined by a physician? Was it:

1. ☐ less than 5 minutes
2. ☐ between 5 and 10 minutes
3. ☐ more than 10 minutes, but less than 30 minutes
4. ☐ 30 minutes or more

(14-19)

A-28

1.b.  How valuable do you feel the physician's examination was?
      Was it:

      1.  ☐  very valuable
      2.  ☐  somewhat valuable
      3.  ☐  not very valuable, or
      4.  ☐  not valuable at all

1.c.  Do you think the Clinic should increase the amount of
      time its doctors spend examining the clinic's patients,
      decrease the amount of time, or keep it about the same?

      1.  ☐  increase
      2.  ☐  same
      3.  ☐  decrease

2.a.  How much time do you recall you spent being examined by
      nurses?  Was it:

      1.  ☐  less than 5 minutes
      2.  ☐  between 5 and 15 minutes
      3.  ☐  more than 15 minutes, but less than 1 hour, or
      4.  ☐  1 hour or more

2.b.  How valuable do you feel the nurses' examination was?  Was it:

      1.  ☐  very valuable
      2.  ☐  somewhat valuable
      3.  ☐  not very valuable
      4.  ☐  not valuable at all

2.c.  Do you think the clinic should increase the amount of time
      its nurses spend examining the clinic's patients, decrease
      the amount of time, or keep it about the same?

      1.  ☐  increase
      2.  ☐  same
      3.  ☐  decrease

(20-24)

A-29

3.a. How much time did you spend being examined with advanced, specialized instruments or computerized equipment? Was it:

1. ☐ less than 5 minutes
2. ☐ between 5 and 15 minutes
3. ☐ more than 15 minutes, but less than 1 hour, or
4. ☐ 1 hour or more

3.b. How valuable do you feel the examination with specialized instruments and computerized equipment was? Was it:

1. ☐ very valuable
2. ☐ somewhat valuable
3. ☐ not very valuable, or
4. ☐ not valuable at all

3.c. Do you think the clinic should increase the amount of time it spends examining patients with advanced, specialized instruments and computerized equipment, decrease the amount of time, or keep it about the same?

1. ☐ increase
2. ☐ same
3. ☐ decrease

4.a. On the day of your visit, how much time did doctors, nurses, and other health care personnel spend explaining their diagnostic procedure or findings to you? Did they spend:

1. ☐ no time at all
2. ☐ less than 5 minutes
3. ☐ 5 to 15 minutes
4. ☐ more than 15 minutes

4.b. Do you think the clinic should increase the amount of time its staff spends explaining diagnostic procedures and findings to patients, decrease the amount of time, or keep it about the same?

1. ☐ increase
2. ☐ same
3. ☐ decrease

A-30

C.  Sometimes the Clinic informs people of its findings by send-
    ing them letters a few weeks after their visit.

    1.  Do you recall receiving a letter from the clinic advising you
        of its findings?

        1.  ☐ yes (go to 2)     0.  ☐ no (END)

    2.  Did you have any difficulty interpreting the contents of
        this letter, or was it comprehensible and clear?

        1.  ☐ difficulty
        2.  ☐ clear

    3.  Did this letter advise you that you had any symptoms which
        might mean cancer?

        1.  ☐ yes (go to 4)     0.  ☐ no (END)

    4.  Did you contact a doctor, clinic, or other health care provider
        because of this letter?

        1.  ☐ yes (ask 5)     0.  ☐ no (END)

    5.  About how long after you visited the clinic do you recall
        contacting the (doctor, clinic, or other health care provider)
        in response to the Clinic's letter?

        Record Number of Weeks

                00  ☐            less than 1 week
                01  ☐            1 week
                02  ☐            2 weeks
                03  ☐            3 weeks
                04  ☐            4 weeks
                05  ☐            5 weeks
                06  ☐            6 weeks
                07  ☐            7 weeks
                08  ☐            8 weeks
                09  ☐            9 weeks
                10  ☐            10 weeks
                11  ☐            11 weeks
                12  ☐            12 weeks
                13  ☐            13 weeks
                14  ☐            14 weeks
                15  ☐            15 weeks
                16  ☐            16 weeks
                17  ☐            over 16 weeks

(30-35)

A-31

6. Did you contact a physician or other kind of health care
   provider?

   1. ☐ Physician (go to 7)
   2. ☐ Other: SPECIFY _____
      _____
      _____
      _____ (go to C.8.).

7. Was the physician you contacted a specialist of some kind?

   1. ☐ Family physician
   2. ☐ Don't know specialty
   3. ☐ Internist or oncologist
   4. ☐ Surgeon
   5. ☐ Other: SPECIFY _____
      _____
      _____
      _____

8. What happened when you saw the doctor (or other health care
   provider)?

   1. ☐ Found I definitely had cancer, and doctor (practitioner)
        began treatment himself. (END)
   2. ☐ Found I definitely had cancer, and doctor (practitioner)
        referred me elsewhere for treatment. (END)
   3. ☐ Doctor was not sure if I had cancer or not, and sent
        me elsewhere for further testing. (Ask C.9.)
   4. ☐ Found I definitely did not have cancer. (END)
   5. ☐ Other:_____
      _____
      _____
      _____

(36-38)

A-32

9. What was the outcome of these tests?

1. ☐ Had cancer.

2. ☐ Did not have cancer.

3. ☐ Went for tests, but never received final diagnosis.

4. ☐ Never went for tests.

5. ☐ Other: SPECIFY _____

_____

_____

_____

THANK YOU VERY MUCH FOR YOUR TIME.   YOU HAVE HELPED US A GREAT DEAL

END

(39)

FACE-TO-FACE INTERVIEW SCHEDULE

## Introduction

People today have many different views on sickness and medical care. It would help us considerably if you would express yourself on some of these matters now.

## Questions

1.  What do you think of physicians in America today?

    Possible probes:

    a.  How do you feel about the care Americans receive?

    b.  Are physicians today any different than in years past?

    c.  Can you recall any experiences to illustrate your point?

2.  Some people believe that medical research in recent years has made great strides in curing patients with cancer, while others think there is little doctors can do for most cancer patients. How do you feel about the ability of doctors today to treat cancer successfully?

    Possible probes:

    a.  Can cure? Optimistic. Can't cure? Fatalistic.

    b.  Other illnesses or just cancer?

    c.  Try to determine extremes.

    d.  How do you feel about medical·efforts to screen for and prevent cancer?

3.  Health care planners in many parts of the country are currently con- sidering establishing screening facilities similar to the Metropolitan Screening Clinic. Is there anything you would care to suggest about how the screening procedure could be improved?

4. Next, we would value your opinion about the methods the Clinic has adopted for detecting illness. As you know, the examination at the clinic employs much specialized equipment. Some people approve of the clinic's reliance on this equipment, while others think it cannot really replace careful examination by a physician.

   How do you feel? (Why?)

   Do you plan to return?

   Possible probes:

   a. How do you feel about the computerized health history equipment?

   b. What about other medical equipment like x-ray, EKG's, and xeromammographies?

5. People respond to feeling ill in many different ways. Some feel it is most important to stay home and seek immediate medical attention, while others think sickness should not prevent them from going to work, attending social functions, or meeting family responsibilities. Which comes closer to your own view?

   Example: last illness. What happened?

   [If retired] How did you behave when you were still working? How often did you stay home with a bad cold? the flu?

6. We would also like to ask about the communications you received from the Clinic and how you responded to them.

   In our telephone interview, you mentioned that you received a letter from the Clinic informing you that you had symptoms that might mean serious illness. How did you feel when you received this letter?

7. After you had read the letter, did you actually think you might have a serious illness, or did you consider it more likely that the clinic had made some kind of mistake?

## NOTES

1. Samuel A. Stouffer, *Social Research to Test Ideas* (New York: The Free Press, 1962), pp. 253–260.

2. See, for example, Renée C. Fox, *Experiment Perilous* (Glencoe, Ill.: The Free Press, 1950); and David Mechanic, *Students Under Stress* (Madison: University of Wisconsin Press, 1978).

# Index

# About the Author

Howard P. Greenwald is a Research Scientist at the Health and Population Center, Battelle Human Affaires Research Centers, Seattle. Formerly, he served as Assistant Professor of Behavioral Science in the Graduate School of Business and the Center for Health Administration Studies at the University of Chicago. He holds a B.A. from the University of Chicago and an M.A. and Ph.D. in sociology from the University of California, Berkeley. A specialist in political and medical sociology as well as organizational behavior, his research encompasses health care, public policy, and problems of the modern labor force. His published work includes studies on the career experiences of technical professionals, the relations between university medical centers and the community, and the effect of human ecology on social organization.